D0687480

Natural Prescriptions For Women

Natural Prescriptions For Women

Robert M. Giller, M.D.
Kathy Matthews

INSTANT IMPROVEMENT, INC.
NEW YORK

This book is not intended to replace the services of a physician, nor is it meant to encourage diagnosis and treatment of illness, disease, or other medical problems by the layman. Any application of the recommendations set forth in the following pages is at the reader's discretion and sole risk. If you are under a physician's care for any condition, he or she can advise you whether the recommendations in this book are suitable for you.

Copyright © 1997 by Robert M. Giller, M.D. and Kathy Matthews

Instant Improvement, Inc.
210 East 86th Street
New York, NY 10028

Editor — Roberta Waddell
Book Design — Gigantic Computing
Cover Design — David Wise

All Rights Reserved

No part of this book may be reproduced by any mechanical, photographic, or electronic process, or in the form of a phonographic or other recording, nor may it be stored in a retrieval system, transmitted, or otherwise copied for public or private use other than for "fair use" without the written permission of the publisher.

Printed in the United States of America by BookCrafters, Inc.

Library of Congress Cataloging-in-Publication Data
Giller, Robert M.
        Natural prescriptions for women / by Robert M. Giller and Kathy
    Matthews.
            p.   cm.
        Includes index.
        ISBN 0-941683-38-9 (hardcover)
        1. Women--Health and hygiene. 2. Women--Diseases--Alternative treatment. 3. Self-care, Health. I. Matthews, Kathy, 1949-   . II. Title
    RA778.G48 1997
    613'.04244--dc21   97-34330

Contents

Introduction

This book is for you as a woman if you want to feel in better control of your health and if you want to live a longer and healthier life. Why a book just for women? All of the other books that I've written have been for anyone. But over the years it's become increasingly obvious to me that women's medical needs are really different and they need special attention.

For too long research studies have been done on men exclusively, directed by the notion that because women's hormonal states fluctuate, they can affect the results of any research. In fact, in 1990, the General Accounting Office issued a dismaying report criticizing the National Institutes of Health for failing to include women in clinical trials conducted to study major diseases.

For years, because of this exclusion of women in clinical trials, they have had less than the best care. For example, there's been less focus on women's diseases like breast cancer and osteoporosis. There's been less focus on the influence of estrogen on functions other than the reproductive. There has been less study of sex-appropriate therapies for disease, like medication to treat heart disease in women that is based on their actual physiology.

Women As Patients

In addition to the obvious differences between men and women, I've noticed other differences in women as patients. They tend to be very open to alternative therapies, very committed to making an effort to adopt different therapies and very sensitive about changes in their bodies. They are also often good consumers and researchers. Many women who come to me already know something about any ailments they have and sometimes they know a great deal.

I recently had a woman patient who was experiencing some menopausal symptoms. As we tried to decide on a course of action, I took a medical history. When asked when her mother had experienced menopause, she answered that her mother had had a hysterectomy while in her late thirties and there was no way to know when a natural menopause would have occurred.

She was mystified as to why her mother had consented to the surgery; there had been no symptoms to indicate it was necessary. Her mother had explained to her that she believed, because she had

had six children and had experienced back troubles, the doctor had simply decided a hysterectomy would be a good solution to any back strain that would result from another pregnancy. Her mother had simply never questioned the doctor about exactly why he was recommending a hysterectomy.

Stories like this remind me how far women have come in taking charge of their bodies and in educating themselves about health concerns.

Women's Particular Needs

Some people have asked me why I would want to focus a book on natural therapies just for women. The truth is, there is a whole range of ailments particular to women that respond very well to natural therapies. Many of these therapies are inter-related and are best understood in the context of women's health.

For example, both men and women have headaches. But many women suffer from headaches as a direct result of fluctuating hormone levels in the course of their menstrual cycles.

Osteoporosis of course is a disease that is a particular problem for women. Heart disease for women must be understood in context — again, in relation to a woman's hormonal levels that change throughout the course of her life. All of these problems, and many others, lend themselves to particular attention.

The Natural Revolution

There have been major changes in the health professions since I began practicing and writing books. In my first book, *Medical Makeover*, written nearly fifteen years ago, I urged patients to take control of their health by making critical diet and lifestyle changes. I was among the first in the medical profession to point to these changes, as opposed to drug therapies, as being the real cornerstone of good, lasting health.

Most people have come around to this view by now. Moreover, the diet and lifestyle approach to maintaining health has grown to embrace natural therapies as a useful component of healthcare. I believe that natural therapies should be a part of every woman's sensible approach to good health.

You are no doubt reading this book because you are looking for another answer . . . one that doesn't involve drugs and surgery for whatever ailments concern you. You are open-minded about healthcare and probably well-read and sophisticated about alternatives to mainstream medicine. But you, like many of my patients, may be confused — confused concerning what to believe about natural therapies and how to proceed when you want to try them.

Today, we are all overwhelmed with information. It seems every day there's a new report on the risks and/or benefits of a treatment, natural or otherwise, for disease. Many doctors are as confused as their patients. Can they in good conscience recommend a natural treatment to a patient? Will it really work?

My Personal Approach

I have used natural treatments with my patients for years. My method has always been to thoroughly research any treatment in a full range of international medical journals. I then work with my patients until, by trial and error, we develop a treatment that is effective.

I have never found the encyclopedia-style vitamin and natural therapy books to be very useful. After all, what matters is what works and, in my experience, some natural therapies simply do not work. Or are unsafe. Or have negative side effects. That is why this book is not an encyclopedia. You may find that some of the natural treatments you have heard of are not included. That's probably because, in working with my patients, I didn't find them to be effective.

I know that, as a consumer, it can be frustrating for you to weave your way through all the claims and counter-claims involving natural treatments. That is why I have written this book. It is my best effort to provide you with what I provide my patients with daily: a thorough, medically safe, proven recommendation on which natural treatment will be effective for your ailment.

As someone who is interested in health and alternative treatments, you no doubt know the reason that many natural treatments are not tested and recommended: money. There's no profit to be made by recommending Coenzyme Q-10 for heart problems. Even though Co Q-10 has been used by health practitioners for decades. Even though it is one of the most powerful treatments for cardiomyopathy available. Even though it increases the survival rate of cardiomyopathy patients tenfold when compared to the combined therapy of ACE inhibitors, diuretics and Lanoxin. Co Q-10 is inexpensive and readily available at your local health food store. But no one is making huge amounts of money on Co Q-10 as they are on ACE inhibitors, diuretics and Lanoxin. There is little incentive for anyone to promote Co Q-10.

Blending The New And The Old

Please understand that I am not a medical heretic; I am not against conventional medical therapies, including surgery and drug treatments. After all, I am a physician who studied for years to learn conventional therapies, and I'm well aware of how essential they can be in saving lives and promoting health. I routinely recommend drugs and surgery when indicated by a patient's condition.

But ever since my early days as a medical student, I have had an active interest in unconventional therapies. As the first American doctor to study acupuncture in China, I had my eyes opened to alternatives to standard American medical treatments. I have always believed that the goal is to cure — by whatever means. Years of experience have taught me that sometimes there's a simple, more natural way.

I've been aware for many years that more and more people are trying to follow a natural approach to healing, but I had no idea how great the public thirst for information had become until I broadcast my first radio call-in show, "In the Doctor's Office," in 1991. I wasn't quite sure what kind of calls to expect from listeners. Of course those who were familiar with my books knew that I specialize in nutrition and "lifestyle therapy." So I certainly expected to get calls from people with questions about diet and supplements and also perhaps about stress reduction, weight loss and exercise. What surprised me was that most of the callers asked questions about very particular problems. They wanted specific solutions to their individual health concerns.

Targeted Natural Medicine

Targeted natural medicine: that's the approach I've taken in this book. Have a good overall daily health regime (see next chapter) and then work on those health areas that concern you.

The first step you take in trying to deal with an ailment should be simple and natural. Natural means can be far more effective than most people realize. For example:

- Both soy foods and the herb black cohosh have been shown to be remarkably effective in eliminating the symptoms of menopause — without any adverse side effects of the sort that can be associated with estrogen replacement therapy.
- The live culture in yogurt — *lactobacillus acidophilus* — really does help cure vagi-

nal yeast infections and may help them from recurring.

- While aspirin may relieve the pain of arthritis, it will do nothing to prevent the progression of the disease. Natural remedies have helped many people find greater mobility and relief from pain.
- The proper nutrients can reverse the results of a Pap smear that indicate the first stages of abnormal tissue growth.
- Quercitin C has been shown to be remarkably helpful to women who suffer from varicose veins by both easing discomfort and improving appearance.

The fact is, natural treatments can be safe, simple, inexpensive and effective. Moreover, they are beneficial to the whole body, the premise being that natural treatments help the body heal itself.

Natural treatments used to be considered suspect by practitioners of traditional medicine. I'm happy to say that is less the case today, especially since the National Institutes of Health have recently funded a department to study alternative therapies. As research has focused more on nutritional causes of disease and as the public has become more responsive to natural treatments, physicians have begun to adopt these techniques.

Many of my patients tell me that their doctors have suggested one or more vitamins and/or minerals for their various conditions. For example, many ophthalmologists now routinely recommend zinc to prevent macular degeneration. Many neurologists recommend vitamins C and E for Parkinson's disease. Little by little these natural approaches are becoming mainstream.

But there is still resistance to changing the way doctors treat disease. Despite overwhelming evidence that some ulcers can be cured — not just temporarily relieved — by antibiotic therapy, there are still doctors who resist recommending this therapy to ulcer patients. Why? It's difficult to change a lifetime of training and, unfortunately, in some cases new treatments are less expensive for the patients, take more time for the doctor to administer and are not paid for by insurance.

What does this mean for the interested patient? You must take charge of your healthcare and be open to new treatments and techniques that have been demonstrated to be safe. With perseverance, you will find doctors who are willing to discuss these new techniques and approaches with you.

Determining exactly what is safe and effective has been a stumbling block when dealing with natural treatments for disease. New discoveries are reported daily. But these news stories are confusing for the public. Frequently the results of these tests are disparaged; sometimes the researchers themselves take a wait-and-see approach. Many women call my radio show simply to ask whether a natural treatment they've heard about is actually okay. This book answers these particular questions and also addresses the more general apprehension many women may have about natural treatments.

The Sources Of My Natural Treatments

The information in this book comes from a number of sources. Once I realized the interest on the part of my radio audience for the latest information on natural therapies, I reviewed all the respected medical journals here and abroad, *The Journal of the American Medical Association,* the *Lancet,* and *The Journal of Clinical Nutrition,* among others, for research published within the past few years that validate particular natural approaches. In most cases, there is a consensus on what works and what doesn't. These treatments have helped my patients. Obviously I can't recommend a treatment that I have not used successfully, even if a number of journals print studies that say it works.

Safety is a major concern in any treatment of disease. Nutritional supplements must be used with discretion. Some patients think that if 100 mg. of something is good, 500 mg. is even better. This is almost never the case. There is no danger in any of the treatments recommended herein when directions are followed as to amounts and duration of treatment.

The suggestions I've made in this book for supplementation are very conservative. Some conditions could require higher doses than those suggested here, but, if that's the case, I feel you should be under the care of a physician who will supervise your condition and I will recommend that in the text. Of course, if you have any question about any treatment, you can discuss it with your doctor.

The Right Approach For You

I've tried to be very clear in this book about:

- when your symptoms indicate you should see a doctor,
- when you can use natural therapies *in conjunction* with traditional methods,
- when you can use natural methods on your own.

I've also tried to be very specific about amount of nutrients to take and for what period of time. I've included recommendations concerning drug interactions where appropriate. I've also included notes at the end of some sections of the book under the heading "In Addition..." reporting new or important treatments that you should ask your doctor about or the latest information on natural treatments that I haven't tried myself with my patients but which I suggest you explore.

I've tried to make this book as close as possible to an actual consultation with a doctor committed to a nondrug, noninvasive, natural approach to healthcare. I believe this book can help you to take charge of your own well-being and allow you not only to avoid illness, but also to achieve optimum vigorous good health.

CHAPTER 1 ———————

A Healthy Woman's Daily Routine

This book is written to help women cope with specific ailments that may trouble them. Many women will simply pick up this book and turn to the subject that concerns them at the moment. I know this is the way most people approach health-care.

But I would like to ask you to do something more. In order to achieve optimum health, you need to follow an overall plan. You can't simply take supplements. You can't simply take herbs. You must pay attention to diet, exercise, and stress control. Many of the diseases women develop in later life (or even at a relatively young age) are the result of neglecting simple basic good health habits that promote optimum health.

As you're already reading a book on natural healing, I know you are probably better versed than the average person about what a sensible approach to good health entails. But you may be leaving out some pieces of the puzzle. Or you may be trying to fool yourself about certain aspects of your lifestyle.

I had a patient, Marie, who was an intelligent and savvy computer programmer. Marie was forty-six years old and working hard to control the effects of an early menopause. She followed a good basic diet, added soy to her food intake, took the various herbs I suggested, cut out sweets and took chromium. But I finally realized that she wasn't doing any exercise.

Marie was clearly embarrassed when I questioned her about it. "I just don't have time, Dr. Giller," she said. "I have a demanding job and a family to take care of and I just can't take an hour or so out of my day to run to the gym."

Marie's problem was common. I can't tell you how many of my patients have "no time" for good health habits. Until they realize what it could cost them in lost time in the future. I'm very sympathetic to Marie's problem because I share it. I have a demanding practice, a family and a wide range of interests that keep me busy outside my office. But I know how important exercise is to my current and future health. So I've managed to wedge it into my busy day.

Habit Exchange

Here's the best hint I can give you about exercise or any other lifestyle change that you are trying to make. You can't change your life overnight. The things you do or don't do every day are habits. If you have ice cream every night while you watch TV or if you never exercise, these are habits. It takes more than a decision to change them.

You need a technique and the one that's worked for me and my patients I call "habit exchange." Don't ever try to change habits, *exchange* them instead. Don't just try to give up ice cream, try to substitute a healthy food. You might just start with fruit or yogurt. Make your focus the new food or treat, and don't agonize about the ice cream you're no longer eating.

The same goes for exercise. Don't decide that you must join a health club or jog every morning. For many people these good intentions evaporate in the demands of everyday life. Instead, try to find something you do nearly every day and see how you can add exercise to it. Maybe you can ride a stationary bike while you watch the news, or walk a few blocks to get your newspaper instead of having it delivered.

I'm always amazed at people who drive around a parking lot for ten minutes looking for a space near the health club! If they simply parked at the far end of the lot and walked briskly to their destination, they wouldn't need a warm-up once they got inside.

Blueprint For Health

What I'm presenting here is a blueprint for optimum health. It gives all the basics that I think are essential to a healthy lifestyle. If your lifestyle is far from what you find on these pages, try to change bit by bit. Remember, you don't have to do it all at once, and every little bit you do will help you toward a healthier future.

Optimum Diet

A good diet is absolutely essential for good health. What you are eating today is going to determine your future health: the bad foods are going to cause chronic disease and the good foods are helping you fight disease and enjoy a longer and healthier life.

> **The diet that will help prevent chronic disease in the future is the same diet that will make you feel better today.**

Here are the six top tips for achieving the best possible diet:

1. Eat Regular Meals At Regular Times.

That means no skipped breakfasts, no late meals, no coffee and candy for lunch.

No matter what your schedule, you should eat three meals daily. I've had patients who are airline or medical employees on erratic shifts, people who work night shifts and entertainers who get up at noon. No matter. I recommend the same to all: shortly after you get up, whatever the time, have your first meal; four or five hours later, have a second meal; usually five or six hours after that, have your final meal of the day.

You need regular meals to give your body a steady supply of fuel throughout the day. Many women who feel tired and irritable eat sporadically. When you've gone without food for six or seven hours, your blood sugar drops and you feel weak, irritable and fatigued. Quick fixes like coffee, sweets or even a cigarette will send your blood sugar soaring and you'll feel temporarily better. But you'll soon crash and need another fix. The toll these highs and lows take on your body is significant, both in terms of how you feel throughout the day and also in its effect on future disease.

Six Critical Good Eating Habits

- **Eat regular meals**
- **Vary your diet**
- **No late meals**
- **No large meals**
- **Prepare in advance**
- **Enlist help**

---

2. Vary Your Diet.

Too many people eat the same thing for breakfast and lunch day after day. I had one woman patient who had eaten nothing but cottage cheese and peaches at lunch for over a year! This practice can limit your intake of crucial nutrients. The more varied your diet, the better your chances of covering all your nutritional bases and satisfying your hunger. Also, when you eat the same thing all the time, you tend not to notice what you've eaten or even that you've eaten at all!

Finally, repeating meals on a regular basis can contribute to food sensitivities. I do a lot of work with patients who suffer from this condition. They have vague symptoms that they never connect with the food they eat. These symptoms can be as obvious as hives but more likely are subtle disorders including fatigue, dizziness, blurred vision, headaches, frequent colds and sore throats, irritable-bowel syndrome and excessive hunger. A varied diet will prevent development of food sensitivities. My basic rule of thumb is try not to eat the same thing at the same meal two days in a row.

3. Limit Your Fat Intake.

Fat is the most concentrated source of calories in your diet. A diet rich in fat puts you at risk for heart disease, our number one killer. A high fat diet has also been linked to two cancers that are major killers among Americans — cancer of the colon and breast cancer.

You can cut down on fat by eating less dairy food, less beef and pork, eliminating fried foods, and avoiding commercial baked items and commercial salad dressings. (One to two tablespoons of olive or canola oil a day can be included in a healthy diet.) If you eliminate the following fatty foods, you'll still get about 20 percent of your calories from the naturally-occurring fat in fish, chicken, tuna, and turkey.

Major Fatty Foods To Avoid

Avocado	Fried Foods	Oils (Except Olive or Canola)
Butter	Ice Cream	Peanut Butter
Cheese	Junk Foods	Red Meats
Chocolate	Luncheon Meats	Seeds
Coconut	Margarine	Shortenings
Cream Sauces	Mayonnaise	Whole Milk
Eggs	Nuts	

Here are some simple steps you can take to cut down on fat in your diet:

- Avoid commercial baked goods that are made with saturated fats and make your own salad dressing with low or nonfat yogurt, spices, garlic, and herbs mixed in the blender.

- Eat more complex carbohydrates, which you'll find in starchy vegetables, whole grain bread, unrefined cereals, brown rice, beans and whole wheat pasta.

These foods should comprise over half your total calories. Carbohydrates are not fattening. They are rich in fiber, which has been shown to help prevent a number of diseases. Carbohydrates are also helpful in stabilizing blood sugar, thereby helping to control your appetite.

4. Increase Your Fiber Intake.

More fiber in your diet can help you prevent colon cancer, lower cholesterol and possibly help prevent the development of heart disease. Fiber also helps stabilize blood sugar, preventing periods of tiredness, irritability and moodiness. And fiber will help you fight constipation.

I suggest you eat more whole grains like oatmeal and bran muffins (but not the commercial kinds which are loaded with fat and sugar), beans in soups and main dishes, fresh fruit as a regular snack and lots of salads with low fat dressings. Also, if you have a particular problem with constipation, take a teaspoon of miller's bran daily:

Some Great Sources Of Fiber:
- Whole Grains
- Fresh Fruits
- Vegetables
- Salads
- Beans
- Cereals

---

5. Shift The Main Source Of Your Protein From Meat To Fish, Poultry And Soy Products, Including Tofu And Soybeans.

Most of us get over 70 percent of our protein from animal and dairy products and most of these foods are too high in fat. Meals based on beans and peas are filling and keep blood sugar on an even keel. Experiment with meatless meals such as a vegetable lasagna made with low fat cheese or stir-fried vegetables with slices of tofu.

6. Avoid Chemical Additives.

Try whenever possible to eat whole, natural foods. Read labels. Cook for yourself when you can, instead of relying on prepared foods.

More Daily-Routine Advice
For Achieving Optimum Health

Sugar

Cut down on your sugar consumption. Sugar not only interferes with your metabolism but can also promote various diseases including tooth decay and diabetes. It also contributes to fatigue, irritability and inability to concentrate, and it makes dieting more difficult. Many of my patients find that when they give up or cut way down on their sugar intake they experience higher and more consistent energy levels. If you eliminate sugar from your diet you'll be surprised at how quickly you'll lose your sweet tooth.

There's sugar in more foods than you think. Learn to read labels and look for the following terms that identify different types of sugars.

Corn Syrup	Lactose	Molasses
Fructose	Maltose	Sorghum
Glucose	Maple Syrup	Sucrose

Caffeine

Many people are addicted to caffeine. While studies attempting to prove that caffeine is implicated in everything from heart disease to high blood pressure have never been conclusive, I believe that the damage excessive caffeine consumption does can't be ignored. Caffeine wreaks havoc on your metabolism and creates a real stress that could precipitate symptoms including headaches, fatigue, irritability, inability to concentrate, depression and nervousness.

Caffeine is a stimulant. After you ingest it your heart beats faster, your blood pressure rises, your stomach jumps, your bowels may react, and your blood vessels constrict. Your body begins to depend on this stimulation. (Indeed, most of my patients who drink coffee have mild to severe withdrawal symptoms when they cut down.) While this stimulation may seem benign, its effect on your body is as if you were constantly in overdrive. It creates a stress that eventually causes mild and major symptoms to develop.

In addition, caffeine can interact with over-the-counter and prescription drugs in unwelcome ways. Birth control pills can slow the elimination of caffeine from the system. Asthma medications may cause excessive nervousness if taken with caffeine.

Caffeine is not found in just coffee and tea. Be sure to avoid medications that contain caffeine (read the label) as well as colas and other drinks that contain it. I suggest you drink no more than one caffeinated or decaffeinated beverage daily.

Patients ask why they can't simply have a caffeinated cup of coffee followed by additional cups of decaf. The point is that you need to break the habit of drinking coffee; many people find that if they continue to drink decaf, they quickly slip back into drinking too much caffeinated coffee. Besides, even decaf contains caffeine in measurable amounts.

> Here are a few food sources and the approximate amount of caffeine they contain:
>
> | Food | Caffeine in milligrams |
> |---|---|
> | 1 cup brewed coffee | 100–150 |
> | 1 cup instant coffee | 85–100 |
> | 1 cup tea | 60–75 |
> | 1 cup decaffeinated coffee | 2–4 |
> | 1 cup cocoa | 40–55 |
> | 1 glass cola (8 oz.) | 40–60 |
> | 1 chocolate bar | 25 |

Alcohol

Cut down, or better yet, eliminate alcohol from your diet. It can cause major health problems as well as social ones. Some people find that a daily habit that began innocently enough as a glass of wine with dinner or a drink right after work soon escalates into a half bottle or more of wine a night, or a series of drinks. It can be difficult to be "moderate" with alcohol; it's safer to abstain.

I do have many patients who are able to drink one glass of wine with dinner and who argue that there are studies demonstrating that this limited amount is beneficial. If you can stick to a single glass every other day, I think it's an acceptable habit.

If you doubt the pervasive effects of alcohol, try abstaining completely for a few days. I promise that you'll notice a real difference in how you feel in the morning and all day long, even if you're a very light drinker. You'll wake up refreshed, without a trace of that nagging morning headache so many who drink learn to live with, you'll have more energy, and you'll simply feel healthier. And, of course, you'll be saving all the calories of alcohol and will probably begin to lose some weight.

Exercise

Exercise is absolutely crucial to optimum health. Its effect on diseases is quite dramatic and there are very few diseases that exercise won't help. I suggest that, at the very least, you exercise for a half-hour, three times a week. This can include a brisk walk, a bike ride, a swim, and so on. Aerobic exercise is best. It increases your heart rate and keeps it elevated for the duration of the exercise.

Stress Control

Stress control is like exercise; sometimes it's difficult to convince someone to do something when they can't *see* results. But it's been proven over and over again that stress control will help prevent and relieve disease. For more information, see STRESS CONTROL, pages 321–329.

Smoking

I've left this until last because I hope that most people who are willing to take charge of their health and use natural treatments don't smoke. If you do smoke, you *must* give it up. There's no point in trying to solve medical problems with nutritional therapy if you are at the same time encouraging all the serious and fatal problems that are caused by smoking. It's like trying to heat a house with all the windows open. There are effective programs to help you stop smoking. For more information, contact the American Cancer Society.

Vitamin/Mineral Supplements

According to a health food industry report, 75 million Americans take a daily supplement, but other people still wonder why they should take vitamins. Can't I just eat a balanced diet? they ask. While I don't recommend megavitamins, I do believe that most everyone needs at least basic supplementation. This will ensure that their body is getting the necessary vitamins to allow daily metabolic processes to function efficiently and to prevent the onset of chronic diseases.

Most people don't eat a diet that is rich or varied enough to supply them with adequate vitamins and minerals. One large study involving 28,000 people showed that more than 60 percent of the people, regardless of income level, manifested at least one symptom of malnutrition. Countless other studies have had similar results.

And remember that the RDA (the recommended daily allowance, which some people argue is adequate for almost everyone) for vitamins and minerals is set at a level shown to prevent the development of serious disease. I think that our goal should go beyond preventing serious disease; I think that we should be moving toward optimum health and should be nourishing our bodies today in a way that will enable them to withstand the onslaughts of disease tomorrow.

Here are two recent reports that you will find interesting:

In a ten-year study of 11,000 men and women at the University of California in Los Angeles, it was found that those who took 300 to 500 mg. of vitamin C daily had a 25 to 45 percent lower death rate from heart disease and a 10 to 42 percent lower mortality from all causes when compared with people who had a substantially lower intake of vitamin C.

In another study, 87,000 nurses were evaluated over an eight-year period. Those who consumed more than 15 to 20 mg. of beta-carotene daily had 40 percent fewer strokes and a 22 percent reduction in heart attacks compared to those who took less than 6 mg. a day. Vitamin E, in doses greater than 100 mg. daily, was associated with a 36 percent lower risk of heart attack than when the amount taken was less than 30 mg. a day.

These are just a tiny sampling of the reports that flood my desk concerning the importance of vitamin and mineral supplementation.

The most exciting recent news about vitamins has concerned the antioxidants. The antioxidants include beta-carotene, vitamin E, vitamin C, and selenium. These chemicals fight the disease and aging processes by acting to absorb the free radicals — waste products of cell metabolism — that act to harm a cell's fragile genetic material.

Antioxidants fight cancer, prevent cholesterol from becoming the sticky stuff that clogs arteries, protect against pollutants, and generally enhance our immune responses. Many studies are showing that people who consume relatively high amounts of the antioxidants experience much lower rates of various cancers, cardiovascular disease and other degenerative diseases.

Help On Buying Vitamins

I feel strongly that you should take a high-quality multiple vitamin/mineral supplement and/or supplements daily. Many people are confused about buying vitamins and this is understandable. There are so many brands and formulations that choosing can be difficult. To simplify matters for you, here's the easiest way to recognize a good quality multivitamin supplement that should save you an afternoon devoted to reading the small print on the back of all those bottles.

Most formulations of a vitamin/mineral supplement (even those with 50 or more mg. of the B's) do not contain enough of the antioxidant vitamins and minerals that I believe you need for optimum health. The amounts I feel are important are 1000 mg. of vitamin C; 400 to 600 I.U. of vitamin E; 10,000 to 25,000 IU of beta-carotene; and 100 to 200 mcg. of selenium.

The Key To The Best Daily Supplement

Your daily supplement should have approximately 50 mg. of the most important B vitamins — B^1, B^2, and B^6. In my experience, a multiple that contains at least this amount of the B's will be well balanced and will also contain a good range of other vitamins, minerals, and trace minerals.

If your formulation does not fall within these ranges, I recommend that, in addition to your daily vitamin/mineral supplement, you take the following antioxidants:

- 500 mg. of vitamin C
- 200 I.U. of vitamin E
- 10,000 I.U. of beta-carotene
- 50 micrograms of selenium

You can buy these supplements separately or you can buy an "antioxidant" formula that should contain these nutrients. Remember that the "antioxidant" formula supplements should be taken *in addition* to your daily vitamin/mineral supplement, not instead of it.

Of course in addition to the supplements I've outlined above, you should also take any supplements recommended in the text to treat any conditions that apply to you.

Many of my patients have questions about vitamins, and here are their common concerns:

Why Are Some Vitamins So Expensive?

Many patients wonder why there is such a great range in prices for vitamins. In general, except for the caveats noted below, you will get what you pay for with supplements. A brand that contains 50 mg. of the B's will probably cost more than one that has only 15 mg. of the B's. In some cases, an expensive advertising budget may drive up the price of a vitamin but an important defining factor in terms of price is the fact that some very expensive supplements are hypoallergenic.

Hypoallergenic supplements are free of the extra ingredients that could cause reactions in sensitive people. If you have known allergies and/or if you notice a reaction that might include headache, nausea, fatigue, palpitations or loose bowel movements within two or three days of taking a new supplement, you may be reacting to an ingredient in that supplement. For example, most vitamin C is derived from corn, and many patients are sensitive to corn products and thus will not be able to take this type of vitamin C. Additionally, many supplements are prepared in a yeast base; some people are sensitive to yeast.

If you notice a reaction that could be connected to a supplement, discontinue any supplements and reintroduce them one at a time at four-day intervals until a reaction signals the problem supplement. Hypoallergenic supplements are more expensive than others but are simply required for some people.

Another factor that affects the price of vitamins is that some are defined as "natural" and this usually means that they cost more. As to "synthetic" versus "natural" vitamins, there is really no difference in terms of the effect of the nutrients on your body. I don't think it's worth paying extra for supplements that are called "natural" as the processing they endure is virtually identical to the processing of the "synthetic" variety and, more importantly, they are chemically identical.

Some argue that the "natural" supplements contain components that are not yet recognized but may be important or even essential to the absorption of that supplement. As of now, there's no evidence to back up this claim and, indeed, there is research to show that some "synthetic" supplements may be more readily absorbed.

Is There Any Advantage To Taking Time-Release Capsules?

Many patients wonder if they are effective. I've never found any independent research which demonstrates that these time-release supplements really work as claimed. I think it's best to simply spread your supplement intake through the day. For example, take your basic supplement with meals (whether you take one or two or more daily), and take your additional antioxidants with different meals. This will help to provide continuing antioxidant protection.

What About Chelated Minerals? Do They Make A Difference?

Patients have also asked me about chelated minerals. Chelation is a process that is supposed to enhance the absorbability of minerals by changing their electrical charge. Again, I have never found chelated minerals to be better absorbed.

What's The Best Way To Store My Vitamins?

As to storing vitamins, you should keep them in a cool, dark place. You shouldn't refrigerate them because the moisture in a refrigerator could damage them. Supplements should be kept in the opaque containers they come in as they are thus best protected from sunlight.

You shouldn't buy huge quantities of vitamins as they will lose potency over a period of time. Some brands of supplements have expiration dates on them, others don't. If in doubt, I suggest you discard any supplements not used within six months of opening.

Informed Prevention

I have one final recommendation. In the course of my studies concerning natural therapies for disease, I have been impressed over and over again by how both genetics and nutrition play a role in our developing disease.

Family history is an important predictor in the development of disease.

At the same time, adequate vitamin and mineral intake can play an important role in preventing or slowing the development of that same disease.

With these two facts in mind, I suggest you take a look at any diseases that you know are common in your family. Whether it's osteoporosis, congestive heart failure, varicose veins or atherosclerosis, make a list of all those diseases which you've seen your mother or father or grandparents suffer from and read about them in this book. (Of course, I only deal with women's ailments in this book so you'll have to look elsewhere for natural treatments for diseases not herein.)

Pay special attention to the natural treatment for these diseases and start to adopt some of those recommendations. With luck you may never develop these diseases but, on the other hand, you could be in the earliest stages of them right now. If you begin to "treat" the disease now, before it has actually manifested itself, I feel confident that you will be helping to slow its possible development.

And Finally. . .

You will notice that in almost every entry in this book there is a notation in the Natural Treatment section which suggests that the supplements are to be taken *in addition* to the basic daily vitamin/mineral you are already taking. If you are troubled by more than one ailment — say, varicose veins, PMS and hypoglycemia — do *not* duplicate any amount of supplements you take.

In other words, if one entry recommends 400 I.U. of vitamin E in addition to your daily vitamin, and another entry recommends 400 I.U. of vitamin E in addition to your daily vitamin, *do not* take an additional 800 I.U. of vitamin E. Never take more of a supplement than recommended in the Healthy Woman's Daily Routine plus a single natural prescription without consulting your doctor.

CHAPTER 2

Acne

Most people think of acne as an adolescent affliction. To a large extent they're right. By age seventeen over 84 percent of American teenagers have suffered from acne and the full range of related mortification and embarrassment. Although acne does not have any serious physical side effects, at an age when a single pimple inspires concern and grief, a persistent case of acne may seem catastrophic.

But teens are not the only ones affected. Acne can flare up in adults as well, just as they're trying to make headway with their careers and relationships. That was the case with my patient Amy.

Amy first came to see me three and a half years ago, after she heard about me from one of her friends. My first impression of her was of youth and high energy. Of an attractive young woman with dark shoulder-length hair and an infectious grin. She swept into my office as though there was not a moment to be lost and held out her hand.

"You've got to help me," she said. "I start a new job next month and I'm getting married six months from now, and I look a mess." She swept her hair back, so that I could see the rash spreading across her forehead and one side of her face.

"If this doesn't clear up by my wedding day I'm going to have to keep the veil down for the reception," she joked, but beneath her small attempt at humor I sensed she was deeply upset.

When I examined Amy I saw that the rash on her face and forehead had also spread along her chest and upper back. She'd had acne on and off since she was fourteen, she told me. Antibiotics helped to clear it up each time, but the last time she had developed a bad yeast infection as a result of the antibiotics.

Now she didn't know what to do. Her new job would be a big step up for her — from installing software she was being promoted to consultant for corporate clients, and appearance was really important when you worked with clients, she told me earnestly. On the other hand, she didn't want to risk another yeast infection, not with her wedding just six months away. Could I do anything to help her?

The first thing we had to do, I told Amy, was some detective work to find out what had brought on her latest acne flare-up.

The Causes Of Acne

The problem is, we still don't know exactly what causes acne, though we do understand its relatively simple mechanism. Acne is a disease of the skin that causes pores to clog and produce pimples on the face, and sometimes, as in Amy's case, on the neck, shoulders and chest.

Acne eruptions occur when the oil glands produce excess sebum, which comes up through the hair follicle to lubricate the skin. Sometimes the excess sebum combines with skin pigmentation to form blackheads on the surface of the skin; other times it blocks the pores beneath the surface of the skin, forming whiteheads. In either case, if irritation causes the follicle to rupture, bacterial infection may produce further inflammation and painful cysts and nodules which can cause scarring if improperly treated.

Severe acne is usually treated with antibiotics to prevent scarring, but, as in Amy's case, long-term antibiotic therapy often results in yeast infections. The yeast infection clears up when the antibiotic is discontinued, but if the root cause of the problem is not addressed, the acne returns.

There's a distinct hereditary factor to acne, which seems to run in families. Aggravating factors include an oily skin, stress, exposure to the sun, and even the changes of the seasons. In adolescence, acne typically starts with a flare-up of androgens, which are the male hormones produced by both the testes and ovaries, and the adrenal glands in both sexes.

Adult women may also experience hormone-induced acne before and during their menstrual period, or they may experience acne as an allergic reaction to food or cosmetics. In my experience, food or cosmetic allergies are the most frequent villains in adult-onset acne.

Amy told me she had no history of allergies, but allergies can develop at any age, so I questioned her closely to get to the source of the problem. Did her acne flare-ups coincide with the start of a new diet? Was she taking any over-the-counter medications? Had she used a new moisturizer, cosmetic, or sunscreen? Was she eating healthy, nutritious food?

A number of interesting studies have shown a direct correlation between acne and diet: people with high fiber, low fat diets have far less acne than do people on high fat diets, probably because dietary fat is believed to cause the production of an excessive amount of sebum, which causes pimples when it clogs the pores.

As Amy went over her routine of the last three weeks, the likely culprit for her latest acne flare-up became quickly apparent. She had been working late hours to clear her desk before going on to her new job, she said. She had been sending out for food, with cheeseburgers and fries heading the list, instead of going home to dinner; sometimes her fiancé would bring a pizza or Chinese food down to her office. "I didn't realize just how much junk food I'd been eating," she said with a sheepish grin.

Amy's Approach

I told Amy that natural therapy would most likely clear up her problem. Certainly further antibiotics were counterindicated in her case. (I have several other acne patients who also came to see me because they were caught up in this cycle of antibiotics and yeast infection.)

I instructed Amy to cut her dietary fat back to 20 percent of her caloric intake, and to try the nutritional supplements that had proven very successful in treating patients with acne. I also urged her to eat lots of fruits and vegetables, and to supplement her high fiber diet with one ounce of an all-bran cereal. The effects of a low fat, high fiber diet supplemented with vitamins and minerals should become evident within three months, I told Amy — not soon enough for the start of her new job, but well before her wedding.

As it turned out, when I saw Amy a month later her acne had largely subsided. There had been no new flare-ups in over two weeks, and she was able to disguise her fading rash with hypoallergenic makeup. "I'm so grateful to you," she said. "I've had the problem for so many years, and now I finally feel I will be able to control it. And that makes all the difference."

Since there is no one single medication that can effectively and safely treat acne, my acne patients are reassured to know that they can control or even prevent the problem with a combination of several natural treatments.

Keep in mind that, just as there are biological differences between all human beings, so there are slight differences between the treatments that work for them. Try the treatments individually or in combination with each other until you find the approach most effective for you.

Check For Potential Allergies

Try to determine if your acne flare-up may have been caused by a food or cosmetic to which you are allergic. If you suspect you know what it is, you should discontinue it immediately. If you don't know, you may be able to look for hidden allergies and identify the offending food or substance through a process of elimination.

Improve Your Nutritional Status

Since dietary fat contributes to the clogging of pores (as well as to many other more serious diseases) it should be cut back to 20 percent of your caloric intake. Make several helpings of fresh fruits and vegetables a daily part of your diet, and supplement your fiber intake with one ounce of an all-bran cereal. Refer to **A HEALTHY WOMAN'S DAILY ROUTINE**, page 19, for additional guidelines on a healthy diet.

Nutritional Supplements For Acne

There are several natural supplements which have been very successful in helping to treat acne when used in conjunction with a healthy diet.

Vitamin A, which is an important antioxidant and which enhances the immune system, is also crucial in helping to maintain a healthy skin and can virtually eliminate milder cases of acne. I prescribe Vitamin A in doses ranging from 10,000 to 25,000 I.U. Since higher doses of Vitamin A can cause side effects, it should be used only under your doctor's supervision.

Vitamin E, which is also an important antioxidant, helps your body absorb and utilize Vitamin A, so I recommend that you take Vitamin E along with Vitamin A.

Zinc insufficiency has been linked with aggravated acne, and several studies have shown that zinc supplements have cleared up the condition. A doctor in Sweden found, in the course of some of his studies, that zinc supplements, taken over twelve weeks, *were as effective as antibiotics or Accutane* in clearing up acne — without the serious side effects.

A selenium deficiency has been linked with severe, or postular acne, and selenium supplements have been used successfully to clear up the condition. The daily multivitamin described in **A HEALTHY WOMAN'S DAILY ROUTINE** will contain adequate selenium for this purpose.

Vitamin B^6 may also be helpful in controlling acne, particularly for women who experience flare-ups around the time of their menstrual period. While some experts recommend taking B^6 the week before and the week after a period, my patients have had better results by taking it every day all month.

And finally, there are the "omegas," which are the essential fatty acids that are proving effective against the inflammations of skin disease. For acne, I prescribe omega 6, found in primrose oil, black currant seed oil, or borage seed.

A Secret Ingredient

Many women have been helped by the use of tea-tree oil in their fight against acne. You can find tea-tree oil, which is the natural substitute for benzoyl peroxide, in your health-food store. Tea-tree oil comes from the Australian native tree *Melaleuca alternifolia,* and also has an antimicrobial effect which helps in reducing acne. It has fewer side effects than benzoyl peroxide, but it takes longer to work, so you have to be patient. You apply it to the affected area every day.

An Acne-Fighting Skin Care Regime

You should notice the effects of the nutritional supplements and low fat diet within a period of three months. In the meantime it is essential that you take proper care of your skin, to avoid additional inflammation, infection, and scarring.

1. When washing, gently does it. Avoid harsh soaps. Use a mild soap such as Dove or Neutrogena, or a cleanser containing salicylic acid which loosens dirt so it can just be rinsed away.
2. Do not squeeze whiteheads which are clogged pores beneath the outer surface of the skin. Leave them alone. They will go away on their own within three or four weeks. Squeezing them can cause infection and scarring. The only time you should

squeeze a pimple is if it's already infected and contains yellow pus, in which case the way to do it is to open the pores by taking a warm bath or shower, or applying a warm moist compress to the area for a few minutes and then squeezing the pimple gently with a tissue until the pus comes out.

3. Remove blackheads gently. Blackheads are plugs of oil that have darkened when mixed with pigmentation or upon contact with the air — they are not dirt, and scrubbing will only make them worse. After taking a warm bath or shower to open the pores, you can remove the blackheads with an extractor, which you can buy at any pharmacy. Do not use your hands or fingernails, as this may cause scarring of the skin.

4. Discourage new blemishes with medicated lotions containing benzoyl peroxide. Since these may dry and redden the skin, start with a 5 percent concentration, which is as effective for many people as the 10 percent version. Apply the lotion to the affected area and about an inch of the surrounding skin, but, to minimize irritation, don't leave the lotion on for extended periods. Apply it in the evening for a couple of hours, and then wash it off before going to bed.

5. If your skin is dry, you can use moisturizer, but make sure that it is hypoallergenic.

6. Make sure that your makeup, foundations and suntan lotions are all hypoallergenic.

A Natural Treatment For Acne

- Modify your diet: eat a low fat (no more than 20 percent of calories from fat), high fiber diet. Eat lots of fresh fruits and vegetables and whole-grain breads and cereals.

- Investigate the possibility of food allergies. If you have no success dealing with this on your own, see a doctor who specializes in nutritional medicine. Once you've identified a food allergy, you must be scrupulous in eliminating it from your diet. You may find that you're allergic to a number of foods or a whole category of foods, such as dairy foods.

In addition to your daily basic antioxidant vitamin/mineral supplement, take:

- Vitamin A: 10,000 I.U. daily.[1]
- Vitamin E (to be taken in conjunction with vitamin A): 400 I.U. daily.
- Zinc: 500 mg. daily.
- Vitamin B[6]: 50 mg. daily.

  Note: Vitamin B[6] is particularly helpful for women who experience pre-menstrual acne flare-ups. They should take it throughout the month.

---

1. Note: See your doctor before taking a higher dosage, or if taking Vitamin A for extended periods.

- Evening primrose oil: 500 mg. three times daily.
- Tea-tree oil: apply topically to affected area once daily.
- In addition you must take special daily care of your skin and follow skin care guidelines given above.

CHAPTER 3 — *Angina*

I've treated many patients for angina, but few made their first visit to my office as dramatically as Celeste, who had been referred to me by her cardiologist. I was on the phone with another patient when my receptionist came rushing in to tell me that a new patient had suddenly taken ill. I strode out into the waiting room and saw a fair slender woman in her early forties bent over in her chair. Her hands were pressed tightly against her chest and her face was very pale, her breathing labored as she took short quick breaths through her open mouth. But even as I reached her side she drew a deeper breath and straightened up. She reached out to show me the small bottle of nitroglycerin clutched in her hand. "I took one of these," she managed to whisper.

Angina is the name of the pain that occurs when the heart is not getting enough oxygen because of an obstruction in the arteries that lead to the heart. The pain, which is normally felt just beneath the sternum or breastbone, may also radiate up to the left shoulder and down inside the left arm, or spread to the back, the jaws, the teeth — sometimes even down the right arm.

The pain is usually described as dull and constricting, but it can be severe, and patients sometimes experience difficulty breathing, along with sweating, dizziness, and nausea.

Angina can be precipitated by exertion — particularly in cold weather. Overeating, stress or emotional upset can also bring it on, as can various drugs such as amphetamines, cocaine, and even oral contraceptives and various anti-cancer drugs.

In Celeste's case, the angina attack had been brought on by her short run from her car to my office on a cold, windy day. Many angina patients who are relatively active in the summer find that the same level of activity in cold weather brings on an attack. She had found almost immediate relief by taking nitroglycerin, a vasodilator which allows the blood to flow more freely by dilating the arteries.

But nitroglycerin only relieves the symptom, not the root cause of the disease. Angina is the symptom of very serious disease of the coronary arterial system, and though many people live for years with angina, it may also be the first sign of an impending heart attack.

Causes Of Angina

Angina is almost always caused by coronary artery disease, particularly atherosclerosis, which is the buildup of deposits on the walls of the arteries. Until fairly recently, it was believed that men suffered more frequently than women from coronary artery disease and womens' symptoms were too often ignored. Now we know that heart disease is the leading cause of death among women and much more attention is being paid to women who suffer from angina.

In addition to nitroglycerin, beta blockers and calcium channel blockers are drugs that are commonly used to control angina. Various surgical procedures such as angioplasty and bypass can also increase the flow of blood to the heart. But there is growing evidence that surgery may be ultimately ineffective for many patients, who experience renewed buildup of deposits a few weeks or months after surgery.

Such was the case with Celeste, who had suffered from angina for two years before undergoing angioplasty to clear out her arteries. Now, barely a year later, she was once again experiencing the pains of angina. She was trying to live as normal a life as possible, she told me, after her examination. I gathered she was happily married and had a seven year old daughter in school. She smiled when she mentioned the child. "I kept putting off getting pregnant, and now I don't know what we ever did without her," she said.

She worked full-time as manager of a department in a retail store, and she liked her job but was unhappy about not being home when her daughter came home from school. "I have a babysitter but a child needs her mother at that age," she said, and when the pinched, anxious look returned to her face I knew she was thinking about her life-threatening illness. "Is there anything you can do to help me?" she asked.

Natural Approach To Angina

I was glad to be able to reassure her. I had been able to help many patients with angina, both young and old, by using natural therapy in conjunction with traditional medical means. Based on my examination and my discussion with her cardiologist, I thought we could effectively reduce the frequency of her angina attacks and perhaps eliminate them altogether, along with the risk of her suffering a heart attack.

Our first goal, I told her, would be to reduce the effects of atherosclerosis, the buildup of deposits on the walls of her arteries. As medical research has shown, and I have found from my own experience with my patients, atherosclerosis can be reversed with a program of diet, exercise, and relaxation techniques.

(For complete details on the program for atherosclerosis patients, please turn to ATHEROSCLEROSIS, page 83.)

I gave Celeste my recommendations for diet and natural therapy, and suggested that, for her exercise, she take up walking several times a week. She could start with very short walks and work up to half an hour or more, providing she had no bad side effects, but I cautioned her against undertaking any more strenuous exercise without supervision.

Finally, I talked to Celeste about the importance of stress management. Few people realize that stress, if badly managed, can be as dangerous to the heart patient as high cholesterol or high blood pressure. We can't avoid stress in our lives, but we can learn to keep its negative impact to a minimum by learning to change our reactions to stressful situations.

I told Celeste that I would like to see her once a month until her condition improved. One month later, she told me she was still experiencing the angina pains. "But not as often, and they don't seem as bad," she reported. "And it makes me feel good to know that I'm controlling the disease instead of it controlling me.

"I've been eating at least five half-cup servings of fruits and vegetables every day, so I'm getting lots of beta-carotene. I guess it's not as difficult as I thought it would be, and my family is eating better as well because of it. I've also been taking Coenzyme Q-10, as well as the DL-carnitine and the fish-oil supplements. Oh, and my vitamin supplements, of course."

She hesitated a moment, and continued. "Another thing. I thought of what you said about stress, and that we cannot eliminate it from our lives. But sometimes we can. The thing that stresses me the most right now is not spending more time with my daughter. So I've decided to change jobs. One of my neighbors needs help in running her store, and I think I'm going to take her up on her offer. It will mean less money, but we'll make do one way or another."

Celeste continued to improve — slowly, with a few setbacks that she refused to find discouraging — and now, nine months later, she's virtually free of the symptoms of her disease. She hasn't experienced an angina attack in almost two months, and she sounds cheerful and optimistic about her prospects.

"I know I'll always have to watch what I eat and drink and do in the future," she said, "but at least I believe I have a future. . .which is more than I did when I first came to see you."

If You Think You Have Angina. . .

I've had many other angina patients who, as Celeste, have seen their life turn around through natural therapy, and I believe that everybody with angina can be helped using natural means and medications under the supervision of a doctor.

If you think you may have angina, you should consult a doctor. For one thing, you may not have angina. It has been reported that up to twenty-five percent of all patients admitted to hospital emergency rooms for chest pains are suffering, not from heart disease, but a hiatal hernia, which is the bulging of the stomach above the diaphragm.

There are also people who thought they had angina but whose pains were due to severe allergic reactions. Osteoarthritis of the upper spine has also been known to mimic angina.

If you do have angina, keep in mind that natural therapy is to be used in conjunction with, not instead of, traditional medicine.

And feel reassured that with certain lifestyle changes and natural therapies, you can dramatically improve the quality of your life, and at the same time increase your potential life span.

Substance Alert!

Smoking takes a great toll on the heart. If you have angina, it is essential that you stop smoking.

Alcohol can have a damaging effect on the heart, and I instruct my patients with angina to stop drinking alcohol.

Caffeine may also be a problem, in that it heightens the blood pressure and puts extra stress on the circulatory system. I tell my patients with angina to limit themselves to one caffeinated drink a day.

Improve Your Nutritional Status

As an angina patient, your goal is to strengthen your heart and promote the unimpeded flow of blood by clearing out your arteries through a healthy diet. Follow the diet in the Chapter on **ATHEROSCLEROSIS**, Page 83. Be sure to avoid fatty or fried foods, as well as butter, cream, and red meat.

Olive oil has a protective effect against heart disease. Don't take excessive amounts of it, but do use it in moderation when cooking, and order dishes made with olive oil when eating out in restaurants.

Eat lots of fresh fruits and vegetables and grains. Beta-carotene, a powerful antioxidant, has proven itself in reducing attacks of angina as well as heart attacks, strokes, and cardiac deaths. The most effective sources of beta-carotene are fresh fruits and vegetables, and I urge my angina patients to eat at least five half-cup servings of fruits and vegetables every day.

Concentrate on the best sources of beta-carotene, which include all yellow/orange fruits and vegetables such as carrots, sweet potatoes, apricots, peaches and cantaloupes, and dark-green leafy vegetables such as broccoli, spinach, kale, and arugula.

Fish oils have also been shown to improve heart function, and are effective in preventing heart disease by reducing dangerous blood fats, in particular triglycerides. I encourage my patients to have grilled, broiled or baked fish as part of their regular diet.

Exercise — With Caution

Exercise is very important for patients with heart and circulatory problems, because it improves circulation while it strengthens the heart. But you must also use basic common sense in your exercise program.

I recommend walking to my angina patients, because it's a simple exercise that does not require any equipment and does not place undue strains on the heart. But if the outside winter air brings on an angina attack, walk in an enclosed shopping mall instead. And if a brisk half-hour walk gives you problems, start out with a slow walk of ten minutes or so. As the weeks go on and you feel better, you can increase the amount and the pace of your exercise.

Nutritional Supplements For Angina

There are several nutritional supplements which have been of invaluable help to people with angina.

The most significant one, when used in the context of an overall treatment plan is Coenzyme Q-10. This supplement is also known as ubiquinone, and has been shown to prevent the accumulation of fatty acids within the heart. It plays a beneficial role in fat and energy metabolism, and is extremely helpful to people who suffer from angina. I'm aware of some reports which claim that Co Q-10 is ineffective, but my patients have invariably found that it reduces their pain and increases their ability to be active without discomfort. I suggest 30 to 60 mg. of Co Q-10 three times a day. You should start seeing results within one to three weeks.

If you're not eating at least five servings of fruits and vegetables rich in beta-carotene, take a beta-carotene supplement daily.

Vitamin E is also important to patients with angina. Low levels of Vitamin E have been implicated in the development of angina, and one study conducted in Scotland revealed that men with low levels of Vitamin E were twice as likely to suffer from angina as people with high levels. In addition, a World Health Organization study found low levels of Vitamin E to be a risk factor for death from heart disease. I believe Vitamin E is important.

Low levels of Vitamin C have also been linked to heart disease, and I recommend daily supplements of Vitamin C.

Selenium is also important to proper heart function, and I suggest that my patients take a selenium supplement.

Magnesium is another mineral that is very important to proper heart function and has been used to control irregular heartbeat. Magnesium deficiencies have been shown to stimulate spasms of the coronary arteries and have been linked to death by heart attack. I recommend a daily supplement of magnesium.

Another supplement that is very helpful to angina patients is DL-carnitine, which is available in health food stores. It improves the burning of fatty acids and improves exercise tolerance by strengthening the heart. In various studies, carnitine has also been shown to be helpful in lowering cholesterol levels and preventing irregular heartbeats. Since carnitine is a substance natural to the body, there is no risk in taking it, and I recommend daily supplements to my patients.

Aspirin, as you may know, keeps the blood flowing freely, and is useful in treating angina. I recommend that my patients take one baby aspirin (60 mg.) a day unless of course they are allergic to aspirin, or have a condition which precludes aspirin, such as bleeding or peptic ulcers or very high blood pressure.

We've already discussed the importance of fish oils for angina patients. I recommend that my patients, in addition to making fresh fish a regular part of their menu, take a Max EPA fish oil supplement daily.

> Though research is preliminary, there is some fascinating material that supports the effectiveness of the amino acid L-lysine, taken in conjunction with vitamin C, in relieving angina. I suggest you try taking up to six grams a day of lysine for a few weeks to see if this gives you any relief.

A Natural Treatment For Angina

In addition to your daily basic antioxidant vitamin/mineral supplement, take:

- Coenzyme Q-10: 30 to 60 mg. three times a day.
- Beta-carotene: eat 5 one-half cup servings of fruits and vegetables rich in beta-carotene including carrots, sweet potatoes, apricots, peaches and cantaloupes, and dark-green leafy vegetables such as broccoli, spinach, kale and arugula. Alternatively, you can take supplements of beta-carotene in amounts of 10,000 I.U. daily.
- Vitamin E: 400 I.U. daily.
- Vitamin C: 1000 mg. daily.
- Selenium: 50 micrograms daily.

- Magnesium: 250 mg. three times a day.
- L-carnitine: 250 mg. three times a day.
- Max EPA: 1000 mg. three times a day.
- One baby aspirin (60 mg.) daily unless you suffer from aspirin sensitivity, high blood pressure or bleeding or peptic ulcer.

Also:

- Include olive oil in your diet when possible and appropriate.
- Adopt a program of supervised exercise. Discuss this with your cardiologist.
- Stop smoking.
- Eliminate caffeine or reduce consumption to no more than one cup of coffee or tea daily.
- Eliminate alcohol from diet.
- Adopt a program of stress management, for example progressive relaxation. (See STRESS CONTROL, page 321).

An Important Notice. . .

Natural remedies will not pre-clude the need for the care of a car-diologist. You should follow your doctor's recommendations con-cerning your care and you should not discontinue any medication without consultation with your doc-tor. All these measures are geared to work in conjunction with a super-vised medical program.

CHAPTER 4 — *Arthritis*

I was surprised to see a youthful, trim woman of sixty in my office a few years ago. I knew that she had asked for an appointment on an emergency basis but she certainly didn't show any signs of traumatic illness. I learned only in the course of a thorough examination that Marjorie was so troubled by arthritis that she couldn't take another day of pain.

Her condition was further exacerbated by her active lifestyle; she was an avid tennis player and enjoyed gardening and playing the piano at family gatherings. All these enhancements to her life were becoming increasingly difficult and even painful and Marjorie was desperate for help.

Marjorie has lots of company; about eighty percent of all women have some degree of arthritis by the age of sixty-five. Osteoarthritis, commonly known as arthritis, is a disease familiar to most people due to years of exposure to advertisements for pain relief.

Marjorie could have been the subject of such an ad. And she was typical in that her hands, hips and back were the primary sources of pain. Arthritis can affect all the weight bearing joints and can strike particularly where there have been previous injuries or surgeries.

The progression of Marjorie's arthritis was also typical: it began with the mildest morning stiffness years ago. As the years went by, Marjorie noticed increasing pain upon exertion. The day after her weekly tennis game would often be spent on painkillers. Gradually her condition had worsened until she found it difficult to perform the smallest tasks and could only get through a brief game of tennis with great difficulty.

Marjorie, like most people, believed that aspirin, or some version of a painkiller, is the major remedy for arthritis. If you have arthritis, you should know that aspirin and other anti-inflammatory drugs treat only the symptoms of the disease, and, in fact, as I'll describe below, they may actually facilitate its progress.

My arthritis patients are always interested to learn that arthritis commonly shows up on an X-ray only after the joint has been affected long enough for it to actually change in appearance.

Often people who feel mild symptoms go to their doctors, complain of stiffness and are X-rayed in an effort to diagnose arthritis. But in the early stages there can be symptoms without concrete X-ray evidence. Thus, if you feel symptoms of arthritis, you could well be in the early stages, even if nothing shows up on an X-ray. In that case, you'd be wise to begin natural therapy right away to prevent the further development of the disease.

Is It Really Arthritis?

Osteoarthritis usually begins as Marjorie's did, with morning stiffness in a joint — perhaps a hip or a hand or the neck or a knee. As you limber up during the course of the day, the pain disappears but, if the joint is overused, the pain worsens. As I mentioned, the weight bearing joints are most commonly affected as cartilage between the joints is destroyed and joints rub against one another. The remaining cartilage can then harden and the edges of the bones develop small growths called spurs that inhibit movement.

After I had diagnosed Marjorie's rather severe arthritis I also had to tell her what I tell all my arthritis patients: successfully coping with arthritis entails real lifestyle changes, but if you're willing to work at it you can live a full and active life.

Six months after beginning my recommended treatments, Marjorie is a new woman. Her arthritis has not disappeared but she can now live with it comfortably. She is relatively pain-free and can enjoy gardening and an occasional set of tennis without severe aftereffects.

As Marjorie says, "It took me a while to find exactly what worked for me. The supplements and the fish oil really seem to help. And the thing about exercise is that I had to learn how to be reasonable about it. I just can't sit for a week and then go out and play tennis like a demon. I have to pace myself. Now I do a simple, modified yoga routine every morning. I try to put every joint through some simple movement. It helps get me going and relieves my stiffness. I used to try to ignore my arthritis. But I paid the price by living in pain. Now, by following some simple guidelines and having a positive attitude, my life is fuller and more fun."

Marjorie is certainly right about having a positive attitude. An optimistic approach can make all the difference. And don't forget to enlist some help from friends when necessary.

One of the most difficult aspects of the disease for many of my women patients is that it is virtually invisible. Though knuckles sometimes become knobby, most women struggle with their arthritis without anyone being the wiser. So while ordinary daily chores can become a challenge, little sympathy is generated and little support comes from friends and family.

My advice is to tell family and friends when your arthritis is troubling you. And tell them what they can do to help. Sometimes a "time out" and some support from a friend can make a big difference in your day.

Treating Arthritis

My goal for arthritis patients is twofold: *you must treat pain while increasing joint mobility.* The traditional response to arthritis is to treat the symptoms with aspirin and aspirin-like NSAIDs (nonsteroidal anti-inflammatory drugs) or ibuprofen, like Nuprin or Advil, or stronger prescription medications. Many people simply take as much of these drugs as they can tolerate to relieve pain while trying to avoid side effects.

The drawback of this course is that these drugs have been shown to inhibit cartilage repair — the very goal that the arthritic patient should hold uppermost. In addition, by masking pain, they can encourage people to overuse joints.

So, while the major symptom of arthritis — pain — is relieved by aspirin and NSAIDs, the patient is encouraging the joint deterioration of the disease by taking them. This surely is a case where natural therapies should play a role in treatment.

Fortunately many natural treatments have proven very successful for arthritis. I encourage my patients to try these suggested treatments. Some will be effective for you while others will not. It really is a trial and error approach. But most all of my patients have found significant relief through a variety of these suggestions.

Improve Your Nutritional Status

If you are a woman past the age of 50, as are most arthritis patients, your body is no longer as efficient at absorbing nutrients as it once was. You may thus have nutritional deficiencies that could be affecting your overall health. For this reason, I think it's especially important for you to be taking a good quality multivitamin daily as described in **A HEALTHY WOMAN'S DAILY ROUTINE**, page 19.

Maintain Optimum Body Weight

If you suffer from arthritis, it is important that you maintain a normal body weight. Excess weight obviously puts a stress on the skeletal system and the weight bearing joints. One of my patients found that just losing 8 pounds and keeping her weight at an optimum 130 made a huge difference in the knee pain that she had endured for years.

In general I recommend that all my arthritis patients follow a good basic diet as described in **A HEALTHY WOMAN'S DAILY ROUTINE**, page 19. It should be rich in whole grains, fresh vegetables and fruits. Try to eliminate as many refined foods as possible, as well as refined sugars, margarine and preserved meats, all of which can exacerbate arthritic symptoms. Avoid fatty foods including fried foods, butter, cream sauces, red meat, cheese and nuts.

Remember that your goal is not only to eliminate substances that might cause symptoms to flare up but also to compensate nutritionally for any aspirin and anti-inflammatory drugs that you may have been taking. These drugs can lead to various nutritional deficiencies by making your body less able to absorb certain nutrients.

The Latest Exciting Arthritis News

If you are troubled by arthritis, you may well have heard news recently about a natural treatment that not only relieves pain, it also promotes the healing of the actual cartilage. This is certainly dramatic news and when I read about it a few years ago I was skeptical. Since then, I've had a number of patients try these supplements with good results.

The supplements, which are available from health food stores, are glucosamine and chondroitin sulfate. The two sulfates should be taken together because they each provide a building block for cartilage in the joints.

European studies have shown these supplements to be highly effective in relieving the symptoms of arthritis, promoting healing and stopping the progression of the disease. No particular negative side effects have been noted.

I should note that these supplements don't work for everyone; some people report no improvement but I've seen enough positive results to encourage you to give it a try. But please be careful to mention to your doctor that you are trying this route. And remember that the substance has not been in use long enough to know if there are any negative long-term side effects.

The Nightshades

You've probably heard about arthritis and the nightshade family of foods. This connection was originally made by Childers, a horticulturist, who found that eliminating foods of the nightshade family cured his arthritis. Dr. Carlton Fredericks popularized this connection between nightshades and arthritis.

While this theory — that long-term consumption of the alkaloids in potatoes, tomatoes, eggplant, peppers, paprika, cayenne, and tobacco inhibit collagen and cartilage repair — has never been conclusively proven, it is true that some patients find relief from their symptoms when they eliminate the named foods.

Studies have confirmed that food sensitivities cause about 5 percent of arthritis and can aggravate symptoms in about 30 percent of arthritis patients even when they are not the cause of the disease. It is well worth eliminating these foods entirely from your diet for a period of a month to see if you find any symptomatic relief. Obviously, if you do, discontinue them permanently. If not, re-introduce them gradually to see if you notice any change in symptoms.

> I'm a great advocate of acupuncture for arthritis and many of my patients have found it gives them dramatic relief from their symptoms, particularly in afflicted hips, knees, feet and hands. You might try it to see if it works for you.

Avoid Artificial Sweeteners

The artificial sweetener aspartame should be avoided by people with arthritis. Aspartame does not cause arthritis but many people who consume moderate or large amounts of aspartame complain of joint pain. If you have joint pain, whether you think it's arthritis or not, eliminate all foods and drinks that contain aspartame to see if your symptoms are affected.

Try Nutritional Supplements

Several nutritional supplements have proven to be very successful for me in treating patients with arthritis. One is the mineral boron. It seems that people who live in places where there is a minimal amount of boron in the soil have a much higher incidence of arthritis. I suggest that patients supplement their diet with boron daily.

The other substance that I've had success with is an amino acid, methionine, which contributes to the creation and repair of cartilage. In one study, it was shown to be even more effective than Motrin in treating the pain of arthritis.

Fish Oil Relief

There's a great deal of evidence that fish oils protect and "lubricate" the joints, aiding in relief from arthritis. The best natural source of course is fish, with herring, salmon, bluefish and tuna leading the list in milligrams of fish oil. I recommend that all my patients with arthritis increase their consumption of fish. In addition there's a supplement, Max EPA, found in health food stores, that contains fish oils and can be beneficial in relieving the symptoms of arthritis.

Aside from the more unusual supplements, there are familiar vitamins and minerals that have been proven to help relieve the symptoms of arthritis and I use them routinely with my patients.

Achieve Optimum Nutritional Status

Pantothenic acid, part of the vitamin B complex, has been shown to help prevent and alleviate arthritis. The connection between this nutrient and arthritis was made nearly forty years ago and researchers are still struggling to come up with a definitive study that shows precisely why it works. But we do know that many people find relief from their symptoms with pantothenic acid.

I suggest a supplement of 3 grams daily, though you'll have to wait one to two weeks before you see any result. If no results are seen in three weeks, discontinue the supplement. Some physicians recommend up to 12 grams of pantothenic acid a day, but this should only be taken under your doctor's supervision.

Vitamin E, because of its antioxidant properties and also because it's been found to inhibit the breakdown of cartilage, is useful in treating arthritis.

Vitamin C, which is important for the synthesis of collagen and the repair of connective tissue, is helpful for arthritic symptoms.

Vitamin B^6 has been helpful for many people with arthritis. Interestingly, many older people are deficient in B^6. The first symptoms of a deficiency include tingling, pain and stiffness in the hands. I recommend that arthritis patients take a supplement of B^6 in addition to the the B^6 that's in your recommended daily multiple vitamin.

One very interesting study found an important relationship between doses of NSAIDs and vitamins B^1 and B^{12}. It seems that in patients with arthritis, administration of these two B vitamins enhanced the effectiveness of the painkilling drugs, allowing for a lower dosage of the drugs. The effect was seen in as little as seven days. If you do take drugs for pain relief, it would be worth taking vitamins B^1 and B^{12} to see if they help you reduce your dosage.

Finally, Vitamin A and the minerals zinc and copper are crucial to the formation of collagen and connective tissues. I suggest that you simply be sure that your daily multivitamin contains at least the minimum RDA of these vitamins and minerals.

Exercise Is Crucial

Remember Marjorie whom we met at the beginning of this section? Marjorie was an avid exerciser, but for someone with arthritis she took the absolutely wrong approach. She pushed herself so hard when she did exercise that the ensuing pain kept her immobile for days.

While I believe that exercise is absolutely critical for women who suffer from arthritis, I stress that moderate exercise is the rule. Women have an advantage here over men. Many men believe that if they don't "burn", exercise isn't working, and the pain of arthritis can stop them from exercising at all.

In my experience, women patients are quicker to realize that regular, moderate exercise can bear fruit in reduced pain and increased mobility. Indeed, arthritis is almost a commandment to exercise; if you don't you will find that your pain increases as muscles weaken and joints stiffen. The "move it or lose it" dictum is particularly true for people with arthritis. But remember that if you exercise too vigorously, you can aggravate your condition and cause pain.

I recommend that all my arthritis patients adopt at least one form of exercise. Pool exercise is really your best choice because it strengthens muscles and increases circulation to the joints without putting any stress on them.

Walking is great exercise for people with arthritis. A simple program that gets you walking briskly for twenty minutes to a half-hour daily is fine. And now that so many shopping malls are open early for walkers, you can't even blame the weather for not getting in your daily half-hour.

Yoga is also an excellent exercise for arthritics. And you might contact your local Y to see if they have any exercises geared for arthritics.

Physical Therapy

In addition to exercise, there are physical therapies that can benefit patients with arthritis. Moist heat and cold packs can provide short-term relief. Sometimes taking a soak in a warm tub once a day can relax the body and soothe the joints.

One of my patients told me that she found a short nap — forty-five minutes did it for her — each day completely rested her body and gave her relief from pain.

A good source for hundreds of items — for bathing, dressing, cooking, etc. — that can make life easier for people who suffer from arthritis is the Sammons Preston Catalog. For a copy, call 800-323-5547

A Natural Treatment For Arthritis

- Lose weight, if necessary, to maintain optimum body weight.

- Improve your diet: eliminate as many re-fined foods as possible and add whole grains, fresh vegetables and fruits. Avoid sugars, fried foods, and preserved meats. Also avoid fatty foods, including red meats, cheeses, cream sauces and nuts. See **Blueprint For Health**, page 21, for more information on diet.

- Increase your consumption of fish, especially herring, salmon, bluefish and tuna, in an effort to add fish oils to your diet.

- Avoid foods from the nightshade family, including tomatoes, potatoes, eggplant, peppers, paprika, cayenne and tobacco, for a month. If you do not experience re-lief, reintroduce these foods to see if they affect your symptoms.

- Avoid the artificial sweetener aspartame.

Add the following supplements and treatments to your daily multivitamin/mineral regime:

- Try taking a combination of glucosamine and chondroitin sulfates. If you weigh between 120 and 200 pounds, you should take 1500 mg. of glucosamine — NAG, N-Acetyl glucosamine is the best form to take — and 1200 mg. of chondroitin per day. Divide the dosage up over the course of the day. You should see results in a month. If no results in two months, dis-continue.

- Boron: 2 mg. daily.

- Methionine: 500 mg. two times a day.

- Max EPA: 1000 mg. three times daily.

- Pantothenic acid: take 3 grams daily for three weeks. If no lessening of symp-toms, discontinue. As I mentioned above, some doctors recommend up to 12 grams of pantothenic acid daily, but this should be attempted only under a doctor's supervision.

- Vitamin E: 400 I.U. daily.

- To enhance the effectiveness of NSAID's: Vitamin B^1: 100 mg. daily; Vitamin B^{12} 1000 micrograms in tablets dissolved un-der the tongue.

- Vitamin B^6: 50 to 100 mg. daily in divided doses (taken in addition to the amount in your daily multiple vitamin/mineral).
- Add exercise to your daily routine. The best choices are swimming, walking and yoga but anything that you can comfortably do and do regularly is helpful.
- Use heat, including a heating pad or moist heat such as a soak in a warm tub, to give relief.
- Try a regular afternoon nap to relax the body.

CHAPTER 5

Atherosclerosis

Atherosclerosis is a disease of the coronary arteries, and is the major cause of illness and death in the United States. It is caused by buildup of a fatty plaque — composed mostly of cholesterol — which narrows the arteries and eventually reduces the amount of blood delivered to the heart.

Since the flow of blood to the heart is not seriously curtailed until the artery is reduced to thirty percent or less of its original size, most people with atherosclerosis have no warning symptoms until the arteries are completely blocked off, and they suffer a heart attack. Such was the case with Ellie Peterson, whose sister May had been a patient of mine for several years.

"I wish you'd see Ellie next time she's in town," May Peterson told me. "I'm really worried about her. They say her heart attack was a minor one, but any heart attack is scary, isn't it, and what's more, she can't seem to get her cholesterol level down under control. They've had her under two different medications, but neither one seems to do the trick. And she tires so easily these days."

At first impression, Ellie, who came to see me a month or so later, appeared both healthy and energetic. She was a short, small-boned woman in her early fifties, with understated makeup and carefully groomed hair.

But the impression of health was illusory. Under the bright lights of the examining room, I noticed the pallor beneath her makeup and the deep circles under her eyes. The fingers of her right hand bore the yellowish stains of nicotine, and she looked tense and unhappy as she sat hunched over, biting her lip.

"Are you still smoking?" I asked her. I knew that her sister had told me she had stopped.

She gave me a rueful smile. "You can tell, can you? I've given it up three times since the heart attack. Right now I'm on nicotine patches, and I've been off cigarettes for over a week. I should have given them up years ago, but there didn't really seem to be a good reason why I should. I knew I had high cholesterol, but there was never any sign of artery disease."

The Telltale Crease

I examined her ear lobes and saw the slightly curved vertical creases on the lower part of her earlobes, believed to be a frequent warning sign of the disease. I pointed them out to Ellie.

The earlobe is dense with blood vessels, and when the blood flow is reduced over a period of time, and these vessels start to collapse, the result is the telltale crease.

Many studies have shown that the crease correlates with the degree of atherosclerosis. The crease is not age-related, though it is more common as we age — as, of course, is atherosclerosis. A crease in your earlobe is not definitive evidence of atherosclerosis, but it is a warning that should be taken seriously.

A physician in Tennessee told an interesting story about a patient who developed an earlobe crease at the age of forty. After following a general fitness program which included walking and nutritional therapy, but without lowering his cholesterol level, the man lost the earlobe crease by the age of forty-nine — anecdotal proof that you improve the health of your arteries by changing your lifestyle.

I examined Ellie and looked at the reports from her internist. I then asked her to tell me about her diet and overall activities. She was eating a low fat diet, she said, and she was taking medication to bring down her cholesterol level, which remained stubbornly high. She had a couple of drinks a day — she had heard that alcohol in moderate levels was good for the heart. She had trouble sleeping and was plagued by numbing fatigue. She didn't have a daily exercise routine, but she had always thought of herself as physically active. She often went sailing in the summer and skiing in the winter — in fact, that's how she had met her fiancé.

"I've been divorced for over twenty years," she told me. "In fact, I raised the kids pretty much on my own. . . there were some tough times. And so, when I met Henry — it was pretty special. It will be the second marriage for us both, but I've postponed the wedding. It wouldn't be fair to Henry, marrying him until I know I'm well. If you can only help me bring down my cholesterol level. . ."

Cholesterol Is Only A Sign

I told Ellie that it was a mistake to concentrate solely on lowering her cholesterol, which is the primary, but not the only cause of atherosclerosis. I explained that cholesterol can only attach itself to an arterial wall if the inner lining of the artery is already damaged.

Once the lining is damaged, white blood cells rush to the site, followed by cholesterol, calcium, and cellular debris. The muscle cells around the artery are altered and they also accumulate cholesterol. The fatty streaks in the arteries continue to develop, thus cutting down the blood and oxygen supply of the tissues that are fed by the blood vessel.

Other Causes Of Atherosclerosis

Most atherosclerosis patients — Ellie among them — don't realize that a number of factors besides cholesterol are implicated in atherosclerosis. For example:

- There's strong evidence that uncontrolled stress promotes heart disease.

- The female sex hormone estradiol, (which is also present in the blood of men) plays a role in the disease. Levels of estradiol are affected by a number of things, including heredity and nutrition, and the higher the level, the greater the odds of atherosclerosis.

- There's evidence that high levels of insulin promote heart disease.

- Research points to a common virus, the cytomegalovirus, as leading to atherosclerosis and heart disease.

- And it's been widely acknowledged that lack of exercise puts more people at risk for atherosclerosis and heart disease than any of the above factors, including high cholesterol levels!

Fighting Atherosclerosis With Lifestyle

I told Ellie, as I've told my other atherosclerosis patients, that she needed to make some major lifestyle changes. It's a mistake to concentrate on lowering cholesterol simply by taking drugs, particularly as recent studies have shown that many cholesterol-lowering drugs themselves cause a higher incidence of death from both heart disease and other causes, including gallbladder disease and kidney failure.

She was not to discontinue the drugs without permission from her regular internist, but she was to take a multi-pronged approach to fighting the disease — the same approach, in fact, that's used for prevention. She was to follow my guidelines for nutritional therapy, give up smoking once and for all, adopt a regular exercise program, eliminate alcohol, cut down on coffee and control her stress.

Stress And Atherosclerosis

It struck me that Ellie was suffering from stress. She had not had an easy life as a single working parent, and sometimes stress itself becomes habit-forming — we lose the ability to shed it. Certainly Ellie's difficulty in sleeping, and the problem she was having giving up cigarettes were both indicative of stress.

Her relationship with her new fiancé was obviously very important to her, but it could also be stressful in itself — it must be difficult to finally find someone after years of going it alone and then find yourself at risk of losing it all.

Ellie lives in another state, and it was two months later, when she came into town to visit her sister, that I saw her again. She smiled widely when she walked into my office, and I saw that she looked much better. Her skin had lost its dull, sallow appearance and the dark circles around her eyes were mostly gone. She handed me her internist's latest lab report.

"My cholesterol count is down from 240 to 210!" she said. "I realize I still have a ways to go, but I never thought I could get it down this far. And another thing. I'm sleeping much better now, and so of course I feel much better. My regular doctor approves, and he's taken me off the cholesterol medications."

Ellie believed that her new exercise program was responsible for her new feeling of well-being. She had started out walking with her fiancé for half an hour each evening before turning in, and had enjoyed it so much that she was also taking early morning walks. In addition, her sister had given her a new exercise bike.

Ellie said she felt relaxed enough these days that she had little trouble in going to sleep, and she even found she didn't miss cigarettes all that much anymore — and that without the benefit of the nicotine patch! She had also cut back on coffee to one cup a day without missing it all that much either.

I congratulated Ellie on her accomplishment — it was indeed an accomplishment, and she seemed happy with herself. But 210 is still too high a cholesterol count, particularly for an atherosclerosis patient, and I told Ellie we'd have to take it down below 200, while increasing her good cholesterol level.

The Other Cholesterol Level: HDL

These days, many people are familiar with the two different types of cholesterol. HDL, the high-density lipoprotein, is the good cholesterol that actually protects you against atherosclerosis. Women with a level of HDL lower than 50 mg./dl — or 40 mg./dl for post-menopausal women — are actually at risk of potential problems even if their overall cholesterol count is normal.

Women with high LDL, the low-density level lipoprotein, or with an overall serum cholesterol level above 256 mg./dl, have five times greater risk of developing heart disease than people whose levels are below 200.

Atherosclerosis And Diet

I questioned Ellie to find out how closely she had followed my nutritional therapy program. She had virtually eliminated all high fat foods, she said, instead of merely trying to count fat calories. She had substituted olive oil for butter in her cooking, and she was using lots of onions and garlic, which her fiancé loved. She was also taking the nutritional supplements I'd recommended.

However, she hadn't included fresh fruits and vegetables in her diet, and once again I stressed their importance in nutritional therapy. Just a few simple additions can make a remarkable difference.

In one study, people who ate just two carrots a day reduced their cholesterol level by 11 percent in just 11 days! (If, for example, your cholesterol is 250, that's a 24 point drop.) I urged Ellie to have at least four servings of fruits and vegetables a day. By doing so, she would also be increasing her fiber intake, which increases HDL levels while decreasing LDL. Fruits and vegetables, I added as a selling point, would be as healthy for her fiancé as for her.

A few weeks after her second visit, Ellie telephoned to tell me that her cholesterol level had gone down further — to 190! — and that she and Henry had set a wedding date.

And then, a month later, Ellie called again. This time, there was the sound of tears in her voice. Her cholesterol readings were moving back up. And she was feeling tired again. And not sleeping well.

It turned out that, in the excitement of making plans for her marriage and new living arrangements, Ellie had given up her exercise program and had virtually discontinued her natural therapies. She was worrying a lot — about her marriage, her health, and even about how her grown children were going to get along with his. In other words, Ellie had given way to stress.

Stress And Atherosclerosis

There have been several studies linking stress to high cholesterol levels and heart disease. People who are stringent about diet and exercise but lax about stress control are still vulnerable to heart disease. And office workers under great pressure to meet a deadline had much higher cholesterol and triglyceride levels than those same workers a few weeks later, after those deadline had been met.

Ellie, scared by her lapse, swore that she would never let it happen again. I didn't talk to her again after that, though I periodically hear about her from her sister May. Ellie, May tells me, is now happily married. Her cholesterol levels have stayed down for almost a year now, and I dare say will continue to stay down now that Ellie had adopted the natural therapies as part of her life.

As I said before, atherosclerosis and it complications are the major causes of illness and death in the

United States, so it is particularly gratifying that it responds so dramatically to natural therapy and a more balanced and relaxed approach to life. Many of my atherosclerosis patients are panic-stricken when they first come to see me after a heart attack, and I tell them they will be fine, because Mother Nature has given them a second chance.

Substance Alert!

Smoking promotes the development of atherosclerosis. Smokers are three times more likely to have a heart attack than non-smokers, and are twenty-one times more likely to die of a heart attack than non-smokers. It is essential that you give up smoking. Even if you've smoked for years, stopping now will immediately help to combat the development of atherosclerosis.

Alcohol can also have a damaging effect on the heart. Though some studies indicate that red wine in moderation can actually help prevent heart disease, the evidence is mixed. While a moderate amount may be helpful, a higher amount is definitely harmful, and elevates your serum cholesterol triglycerides and your uric acid levels. Your blood pressure may also be increased. My advice is to eliminate alcohol completely.

Caffeine may also be a problem, in that it increases blood pressure and puts extra stress on the circulatory system. I recommend you limit yourself to one caffeinated drink a day.

Exercise Is Essential

Since sedentary living is the major cause of fatal heart attacks, the first and most important step of your natural therapy program is regular exercise. Regular exercise strengthens the heart muscle, reduces blood pressure, regulates blood sugar levels, lowers body weight and reduces stress. It also raises levels of HDL, the good cholesterol, while lowering LDL, the damaging cholesterol.

You don't need to join a gym, or undertake a complicated exercise program. Just walking briskly for half an hour several days a week will bring desired results. Many of my patients who gave up on gyms or complex exercise equipment found that they could easily fit walking into their daily schedule.

If you're out of shape, you can start with shorter sessions and work up to more. There are many excellent books on how to develop your own exercise program which will help you to develop one tailored to your endurance and needs.

Stress Control Techniques

Most women have a great deal of stress in their lives. They cannot eliminate the stress, but they can control their responses to stressful outside stimuli. Exercise will help, and there are various other stress control techniques, from meditation to yoga. I recommend that you experiment with various methods until you find the one best suited to you. See STRESS CONTROL, page 321 for detailed information on coping with stress.

Stress isn't always limited to outside stimuli. You can actually cause your own stress when you get angry. A recent study in the *American Journal of Cardiology* found that when people with heart disease get angry, the pumping efficiency of their hearts drops by five percentage points. In fact, hostility is a stronger predictor of death than other factors, including smoking, high blood pressure, and high cholesterol. You can't completely eliminate anger, but by being aware of it and using stress control techniques you can mitigate the danger of anger to your heart.

Improve Your Nutritional Status

As an atherosclerosis patient, your goal is to strengthen your heart and promote the unimpeded flow of blood by clearing out your arteries through a healthy diet.

You may have been told to eat a low fat diet, but, instead of counting fat calories, it's better to eliminate or cut way back on all high fat foods. These include all red meat, cheese (other than skim cottage cheese), eggs, cream sauces, nuts, chocolate, ice-cream, butter, margarine, mayonnaise and avocado. Use olive oil instead of butter or margarine.

Avoid all fried foods.

Cut down on sugar intake. Most people don't realize that sugar affects cholesterol and stimulates insulin production, which in turn increases triglycerides, another fat in the blood which promotes heart disease.

Eat lots of fruits and vegetables. Beta-carotene, a powerful antioxidant, has proven itself in reducing attacks of angina as well as heart attacks, strokes, and cardiac deaths. The most effective source of beta-carotene is fresh fruits and vegetables, and I urge my patients to eat at least five half-cup servings of fruits and vegetables every day. Concentrate on the best sources of beta-carotene, which include all yellow/orange fruits and vegetables such as carrots, sweet potatoes, apricots, peaches and cantaloupes, and dark-green leafy vegetables such as broccoli, spinach, kale, and arugula.

Fish oils have also been shown to improve heart function, and are effective in preventing heart disease by reducing dangerous blood fats, particularly triglycerides. I encourage my patients to have grilled, broiled or baked fish as part of their regular diet.

Nutritional Supplements For Atherosclerosis

As I mentioned earlier, the fatty plaques that are the cause of atherosclerosis accumulate on arterial walls that were previously damaged. How does that damage occur? Evidence points to free radicals as the culprits. Free radicals are the highly reactive substances all around us: in tobacco smoke, radiation, herbicides, chemical fertilizers and polluted air. Our own bodies also manufacture free radicals during the normal metabolic process. Free radicals, which make metals rust, make fruit spoil and oil go rancid also damage the cells of our body and undermine their regular activities.

Antioxidant supplements are our primary defense against free radical attack. Vitamins C, E, beta-carotene and selenium are the key antioxidants that inactivate the free radicals in our body. An interesting study found that a high level of antioxidants in the blood is a more accurate predictor of your health than are blood pressure or cholesterol levels. Another eight year study showed that people who take daily doses of vitamin E appear to cut their risk of heart disease from one-third to one-half. I recommend antioxidants to all my patients. Women who are striving to control or reduce atherosclerosis should take even greater amounts.

Another nutrient that has shown itself to be effective in the prevention and treatment of atherosclerosis is vitamin B^6, or pyridoxine. Vitamin B^6 is believed to control a substance that damages the cells of the arterial walls. It also inhibits clotting, or platelet aggregation, which inhibits the flow of blood through the circulatory system.

Coenzyme Q-10, also known as ubiquinone, has also been shown to prevent the accumulation of fatty acids in the heart, and plays a beneficial role in fat and energy metabolism.

Magnesium is a mineral that is essential to heart function, and deficiencies of magnesium stimulate spasms of the coronary arteries, and have been linked to increased rates of heart attack. Furthermore, magnesium increases levels of HDL and decreases platelet aggregation and clotting. In one interesting study, people who had adequate magnesium in their water supply were found to have less heart disease than people who didn't. I think that magnesium supplementation is an absolutely critical approach for control of atherosclerosis.

Carnitine, an amino acid, improves the burning of fatty acids and improves the heart's tolerance for exercise. It also increases HDL levels while decreasing triglyceride and cholesterol levels.

As I said earlier, fish oils or omega-3 oils are helpful in preventing atherosclerosis. Eskimos and the Japanese, who eat diets high in fish oils, have significantly less cardiovascular disease. While the best source of fish oils is fish, I also recommend that you take a Max EPA supplement.

I also recommend the mineral chromium, which helps stabilize sugar and raises the levels of HDL cholesterol.

A Natural Treatment For Atherosclerosis

- Reduce all fats in the diet, particularly cholesterol-rich foods including red meat, cheese, eggs, cream sauces, nuts, milk, chocolate, ice cream, butter, margarine, mayonnaise and avocado.
- Eliminate fried foods entirely.
- Reduce sugar intake.
- Eliminate caffeine consumption or cut down to one caffeinated drink daily.
- Eat at least four servings of fresh fruits and vegetables daily.

- Increase fiber intake. Oat bran cereal at breakfast is a good way to do this.
- Use onions liberally in cooking.
- Use garlic liberally in cooking and/or take garlic capsules: one capsule three times daily.
- Adopt a regular exercise program. Walking three times a week for a half-hour is a good beginning.
- Stop smoking.
- Eliminate alcohol.
- Control stress and work particularly hard to control anger (see STRESS CONTROL, page 321).

In addition to your daily basic antioxidant vitamin/mineral supplement, take:

- Vitamin C: 1000 mg. daily.
- Vitamin E: 400 I.U. daily.
- Beta-carotene: 10,000 mg. daily.
- Selenium: 50 micrograms daily.
- Vitamin B^6: 100 mg. daily.
- Coenzyme Q-10: 30 to 60 mg. three times daily.
- Magnesium: 250 mg. three times daily.
- Carnitine: 250 mg. three times daily.
- Max EPA: 1000 mg. three times daily.
- Chromium: 100 micrograms twice daily.

If your cholesterol is high, take:

- Niacin: 1500 mg. daily of the "no flush" variety.

Also:

- Increase your consumption of fish, particularly salmon.

CHAPTER 6

Back Pain

Susan had been my patient for a few years. In her mid-fifties and in good general health, she had originally come to see me for help in losing weight and when her weight-loss goal had been reached (she had shed nearly twenty pounds and kept them off!) she continued to see me for the occasional ailment.

Her call on Monday morning surprised me: "Dr. Giller, I think I've broken my back." Susan explained that she was phoning from bed; immobilized, she had awakened in the morning and was unable to get up. Her back pain was extreme.

The day before she had helped her daughter move into a new apartment. Though she couldn't recall lifting anything extraordinarily heavy, she had done lots of bending and twisting as she unpacked boxes and reached to store things on high shelves. She was certain that these chores had broken her back and her severe pain was a delayed reaction.

If you have ever suffered from back pain, you'll recognize Susan's story. Of course she had not broken her back. She was simply feeling the most difficult and painful symptom of perhaps our nation's leading cause of work absenteeism and general discomfort.

Back pain is almost as common as the common cold in keeping people from work, keeping them from activities they enjoy and keeping them generally uncomfortable and sometimes in serious pain. Four out of five Americans will experience back pain at some point in their lives. Half of these people find that back pain becomes a recurring affliction.

Some people suffer an occasional backache after they do too much yard work; some women get a backache every month with their period; some people get a backache after an all-day car ride. These backaches have obvious causes. Usually a bit of rest, an aspirin or a simple pain reliever and perhaps a heating pad solve the problem.

But the people who often complain to me are those who have chronic "bad backs". That is, they feel fine most of the time but then, seemingly out of the blue, their lower back will begin to ache. Sometimes they're under particular stress or perhaps they just moved in an odd way when they got into the car.

Sometimes, as in Susan's case, they can point to a particular event that precipitated the pain but often they can't. Sometimes the pain is so bad they have to go to bed. Sometimes the pain lasts for a day; sometimes they'll have an episode of pain that will last for a few weeks; sometimes they'll experience pain for a period of a month or two.

Women And Back Pain

Women can be particularly vulnerable to chronic back pain. Pregnancy and childcare take a toll on a woman's backs. I had a patient who was caring for three children under the age of five. She carried one in a backpack and often wheeled the two others around in a double stroller. She was constantly bending and lifting increasingly heavy children and she had no time for exercise. And she couldn't understand why she had chronic back pain!

Many women have weak abdominal muscles — the muscles that hold the back in correct alignment — and at the same time they have insufficient upper body strength. They rely upon their backs when they need to pick something up and eventually the back rebels.

An Important Note. . .

Before I say any more about back pain, I should tell you that, if you have severe pain, pain that lasts for more than several days, or weakness or tingling in your legs and feet, you should consult a doctor. Back problems that are caused by congenital deformities or severe injuries will need the care of a physician. But if you have occasional or even regular general pain you probably can rid yourself of that pain by following some basic rules and adopting a simple exercise program.

I've found over the years that one of the biggest challenges in controlling back pain is convincing the patient that simple measures, if adopted consistently, really will make a difference.

> There is an anti-inflammatory drug, colchicine, that seems to be helpful in relieving back pain for some people when injected intravenously. It often takes at least four injections over a period of time to be effective.
>
> If natural treatments are not successful, you might discuss colchicine with your doctor.

Fortunately, when Susan came in for an examination, no structural disorder was found. While she had feared that surgery would be her only option (her sister had had spinal surgery and still suffered occasional pain), she was thrilled to learn that a natural approach could save her from surgery and also permanently eliminate her pain. Though she had to start slowly with mild exercises, within three weeks she called to report that her pain was virtually gone.

Why Your Back Hurts

The back is a finely tuned instrument and its proper functioning depends on a complex system of muscles, ligaments and bones — those of the spine itself — to work. The backbone is, in effect, a collection of more than thirty bones that are lined up like spools on a rod. The vertebra — the "spool" bones — are separated by a spongy pad called a disc. The disc acts as a shock absorber.

The term "slipped disc" is misleading: a disc never slips but it sometimes bulges out and presses against a nerve in the spine, causing pain. Most pain in the lower back is caused by strained and torn muscles, ligaments and tendons.

Disc injury, which is less common, can be more serious. Sometimes the muscles that surround the injured back can go into spasms which effectively immobilize the back (it seems to be nature's way of preventing further movement) and can also be severely painful.

If you have pain that radiates down your leg, this is known as sciatica and it's caused by irritation of the sciatic nerve — usually due to pressure from a disc.

If your back is causing you severe pain, you should see a doctor for an evaluation. Just remember that, in many cases, natural remedies will work as well as medications or surgery.

Your First Step For Back Pain

What do you do when you suddenly feel that major ache in your back? If you're feeling discomfort, the best thing may be to take aspirin or an NSAID like ibuprofen to relieve pain. If you have a history of acid indigestion, heartburn, or ulcer symptoms, acetaminophen is the preferred pain reliever. (Just remember that the use of pain relievers should be for the short term only. I recently had a patient who had taken so much ibuprofen to relieve his back pain that he suffered kidney damage. Fortunately, the damage was not permanent. NSAID's can also irritate the stomach and exacerbate an ulcer.)

In addition, it's very helpful to take 1200 mg. of calcium to help relax your back. Then you need to rest your back. This is best done in bed with your knees raised.

> **Many of my patients have found great relief from back pain with the help of acupuncture. This does not supplant the need for regular exercise but it can help relieve pain and inflammation and make daily activity, including exercise, easier.**

While you are resting your back you can begin simple stretching exercises: with one leg flat on the bed pull the other bent knee to your chest. Hold it there for a few seconds and then release it and repeat with the other leg. This is an exercise that you should do regularly if you have a troublesome back.

Exercise, Exercise, Exercise. . .

While you may need time to rest a back when you feel initial pain, too much bedrest is actually counterproductive. Resting muscle fibers start to shorten and stiffen within days and as little as two weeks of bed rest can cause demineralization of your bones, and their return to normal can take many months.

A day or two should be the most time you should spend immobilized. As soon as you feel able, you should start moving and begin the crucial exercises that will help you heal your back and avoid future problems. I really believe that the key to a strong, healthy back is movement. Regular, correct movement will relieve pain, get you strong and keep you healthy.

Marianne, a graphics designer, is one of my patients who has learned to conquer her back problems. Here is how she describes her backaches: "My back got really bad after my third baby. I'd always had occasional back twinges before that but nothing I couldn't live with. But after my daughter was born, my back would go into spasms about every couple of months. I'd have to lie in bed for days until I could move again. Needless to say, with three children, this wasn't easy.

"Sometimes I'd feel pain for weeks at a time and it affected every minute of my day. I'd get impatient with the kids and I always felt tired because that ache was always there in the background.

"But now that I know how to treat my back I haven't had an ache in two years. I always knew I should do exercises for my back but I just never did. Now I do them every morning. They're simple and they take almost no time. I do back stretches, bent-knee sit-ups and some pelvic tilts. That's it.

"Of course I'm careful about lifting and how I move and bend, and I'm very careful about stretching regularly when I'm working at my desk, but the relief of not having weeks of distracting pain is well worth the few minutes it takes every morning to do the exercises."

Many people with back problems are aware that exercises might help but they don't do them. I can't tell you how many patients have told me that they stopped back exercises because they seemed so simple they didn't believe they could really be making a difference and, besides, their back was feeling OK.

The truth is, exercises make all the difference and they can help you banish back pain entirely. The key to avoiding back problems is developing strong limber muscles in the lower back and also in the abdomen.

The Best Basic Back Exercises

I've already mentioned the simple stretch you can do in bed, even if you're feeling pain. Here are the other three exercises that you should do at least once, and probably twice, a day:

Bent-Knee Sit-Ups

Lie on your back with your knees bent. With your arms extended toward your knees, do a sit-up. It is not necessary to actually sit up; in fact you should simply lift your head and shoulders off the floor. You'll feel the pull in your stomach. You should do twenty-five of these. When your stomach muscles are strengthened, you can cross your arms in front of your chest as you do the sit-up.

Pelvic Tilt

Lie on the floor and tilt your pelvis so that the small of your back is flattened into the floor. Press your back down while counting to ten. Repeat this exercise ten times.

There is one more important exercise to do and I suggest that you do it throughout the day.

Wall Tilt

Stand about ten inches from a wall. Bending your knees, let your back rest against the wall (use your hands to guide you back so your back muscles won't strain). As in the pelvic tilt, press the small of your back hard into the wall, feeling the stretch in both your back and in the front of your thighs. Hold for a count of ten. Repeat two or three times.

This last wall press exercise is very effective in stretching your back and in relieving pain. It's particularly useful if you work at a desk or in a sitting position. Most people aren't aware that sitting is the position that's hardest on the back. Even if you sit correctly in a well-designed chair, the pressure on your discs is twice as much as when you stand.

And when you lie down, the pressure is half what it is when you're standing. If you sit for long periods, it's essential that you take frequent breaks. I suggest to my patients with back problems that they break for a back stretch every half-hour. Stand up, do a wall tilt or two, stretch your arms and your neck.

And More Exercise

In addition to the crucial back exercises described above, it's important that someone with a back problem get regular exercise that works the whole body. The best activities, considering back pain, include swimming, cycling (providing you cycle in an upright position), walking (probably the best overall exercise for people with back problems), and rowing (if you are scrupulous about maintaining a straight back).

Activities that are riskier because of back twisting and jarring include jogging, golf, tennis, bowling, football, basketball, baseball and weightlifting.

Other Natural Approaches To Back Pain

Obesity can be a major factor in back problems. It stands to reason that a back which is carrying excessive weight can readily become strained. If you are overweight, you need to reduce.

Nutrition is important in maintaining a healthy back and certain supplements can help relieve pain and strengthen tissue. I suggest that you be sure to take Vitamin C. In addition, calcium at bedtime to relax muscles is helpful.

If you have been told that your back pain is associated with arthritis, the fish oil supplement, Max EPA can be beneficial.

There are many tips that can help you with your everyday movements for times when your back is in pain and also to simply help you relieve back stress. I'll list them below at the end of the Natural Prescription for Back Pain.

A Natural Treatment For Back Pain

- If you are in severe pain, if you feel tingling in your legs or feet, if your backache is due to a congenital deformity or an injury, you should consult with a doctor. You may still be able to heal your back yourself with the exercises below but you should confirm that nothing serious is wrong with your back first.

- If you're feeling pain in your back, try to rest it. If necessary, rest in bed. Take 1200 mg. of calcium to relax your back. Do the knee-to-chest exercise described above, alternately lifting one knee to your chest, keeping the other flat on the bed. Do this every half-hour or so while resting in bed.

- Do the exercises described above every morning and every evening. There are four basic exercises: the knee stretch, the bent-knee sit-up, the pelvic tilt and the wall tilt. You must do them religiously if you want to enjoy their benefits. Don't do any strenuous exercise first thing in the morning.

- When severe pain is improved, get regular aerobic exercise such as walking, cycling, etc.

- If you sit for long periods of time, you must take regular breaks that include doing the wall tilt described above and overall stretching. Take a break every half-hour. This includes stopping while on long car rides or getting up on plane rides to stretch.

- If you are overweight, you must lose weight to lessen the strain on your spine.

In addition to your daily basic antioxidant vitamin/mineral supplement, take:

- Vitamin C: 500 mg. three times a day with meals.
- Calcium: 1200 mg. at bedtime.
- Vitamin E: 400 I.U. daily.
- Max EPA: 1000 mg. three times daily if you have been told you have arthritis that contributes to your back pain.

**Here are some tips on back-wise ways
to get through your day:**

- Pay attention to your posture: stand with your back flat, your pelvis tucked under and your knees relaxed. Avoid any position that puts your back in a swayback position.
- Never bend with the knees straight; always lift using your leg muscles, not your back muscles.
- Carry heavy objects close to your body.
- When you work standing up, such as at a sink, rest your foot a few inches from the floor, say, on the floor of the base cabinet. This keeps your pelvis tucked in rather than swaybacked.
- When sitting, try to keep your knees higher than your hips, by resting them on an ottoman or a pile of books. This is especially important if you spend long periods of time sitting.
- Keep your car seat close to the steering wheel so your lower back is flattened and you're not leaning forward.
- Try not to sleep on your stomach and if you must, try using a pillow under your hips to prevent your back from being in a swayback position.
- Never bend forward without bending your knees and tucking your buttocks under.

CHAPTER 7

Candidiasis

Candida albicans is a yeast that is always present in our gastrointestinal tracts. It's kept in check by the friendly bacteria that also inhabit our systems. But when we take antibiotics for a bacterial infection, they kill the friendly bacteria along with the harmful bacteria, and the candida yeast is free to proliferate wildly. Other medications connected with the growth of candida yeast are oral contraceptives, corticosteroids, and drugs used for ulcers, such as Tagamet or Zantac. Even too much sugar in the diet encourages the growth of the candida yeast.

A woman who is on birth control pills, eats a lot of sugar, and has had a few courses of antibiotics is at high risk of developing candidiasis, and women with diabetes are also at risk, because the environment of their vagina is conducive to the growth of the yeast.

Once the candida yeast starts growing out of control, all sorts of symptoms and ailments begin to develop. Frequent vaginal infections are an indication of candidiasis. Other problems due to candidiasis include thrush, which is candida overgrowth of the mouth, canker sores, coughing and a sore throat, bloating and gas, constipation, rectal itch, cramps, bladder infections, fatigue and a loss of interest in sex, allergies, depression, and an inability to concentrate.

To make matters worse, candidiasis also depresses the immune system, making the body vulnerable to infection. This is often the beginning of the classic vicious cycle: the more infections you succumb to, the more antibiotics you take, and the more antibiotics you take, the more you are apt to develop candidiasis, which is conducive to additional infections.

Misunderstood Candida

A major problem to date has been that many doctors don't recognize or acknowledge candidiasis, but treat only its various side effects, such as thrush or vaginal infections, without recognizing their common root cause. In fact, a number of years ago there was an article in *The New England Journal of Medicine* which claimed that there is no such thing as candidiasis. But the overwhelming criticism of the article by various physicians, who pointed out its poor methodology and scorned its conclusions, convinced me that there are many other physicians who are well familiar with the multiple manifestations of the syndrome.

One of the women who had gone from one physician to the other for various problems caused by candidiasis is a television producer I'll call Tracy. She said she'd been treated twice for yeast infections during the past year, and in addition she'd been having chronic intestinal problems such as bloating, gas, and cramps. But the worst thing for someone in her high-energy business was that she felt tired all the time, often unable to concentrate. "I'm not performing up to par, and I'm afraid it's hurting my career," Tracy told me.

Though many patients with candidiasis are on, or have just finished, a long antibiotic course, Tracy had not been taking antibiotics. She did say, however, that she'd been on the birth control pill for seven years. Also, since she didn't have to worry about her weight, she tended to eat a lot of cookies and candies, which gave her a quick jolt of energy.

After I diagnosed her candidiasis, Tracy agreed to go off the birth control pill and use an alternative method of birth control. I explained that she could go back on the pill when the candidiasis had cleared up, but, if there were another flare-up, I recommended she go off the pill permanently.

Candida And Diet

I then told Tracy that the most effective way to fight candidiasis was to modify her diet. Candida yeast does not thrive in an yeast-free, sugar-free intestinal environment, so I advised Tracy to give up all foods containing yeast and sugar. I also told her that garlic is an effective antifungal agent, and recommended that she add fresh garlic to her diet, or take it as a supplement in the form of capsules. And, to maintain the friendly bacteria that fight candida yeast, I recommended that she add yogurt to her diet, or start taking regular acidophilus supplements. Finally, I told her about caprylic acid, which is a naturally-occurring fatty acid that is helpful in fighting candidiasis.

After the first week on the yeast-free, sugar-free diet and the natural supplements, Tracy called to tell me how much better she felt. "I haven't had any more of those cramps or that awful bloating," she told me, "and I'm even beginning to feel less tired. I've been exhausted for so long, from the moment I get out of bed in the morning, that I hardly remember what it's like to wake up feeling alive."

Two months later, when Tracy felt that her candidiasis had completely cleared up, she went back on the pill, but decided to stay on a low-yeast and low-sugar diet. "I feel so much better now," she told me "that I don't want to risk a relapse. Oh, I'll have the occasional piece of French bread, or a cookie after dinner, but I no longer have the obligatory Danish pastry with my morning coffee."

Tracy's recovery from candidiasis was swift. She was so eager to rid herself of the infection that she had wasted no time in discontinuing the pill and modifying her diet.

Even patients on long term antibiotics can reduce candida, and modify its side effects, by curtailing their diet. One of them was Joan, a landscape designer who spends a great deal of time outdoors, and who was taking antibiotics for a particularly resistant case of Lyme's disease at the time she developed candidiasis.

Since there could be no question of her discontinuing antibiotics until the Lyme infection was under control, I told Joan to follow the same diet and take the same supplements Tracy had been taking. In fact, since Joan had to take antibiotics three times a day, I suggested that she take the supplement of acidophilus at the same time, to decrease the chance of forgetting. Within a week, Joan too reported that her digestive problems had almost cleared up, as had the white coating on her tongue and her allergic rashes.

A Natural Treatment For Candidiasis

- If possible, after consultation with your doctor, eliminate antibiotics, birth control pills, corticosteroids and ulcer drugs.
- Begin a yeast- and sugar-free diet and follow it strictly for at least ten days. If your symptoms diminish, you know that you have been suffering from candidiasis.

  Depending on the severity of your symptoms, you'll have to follow the yeast-free diet for three to twelve months. Eliminate the following foods from your diet: bread, baked goods, cheese, mushrooms, vinegar, soy sauce, fermented foods, alcohol. Also eliminate sugar, including all sweets: cookies, candy, ice cream, soda, diet soda, dried fruit, chocolate and sweeteners, including fructose, malt, barley and fruit juice.

In addition to your daily basic antioxidant vitamin/mineral supplement:

- Add lactobacillus acidophilus to your diet in natural form in yogurt (make sure the yogurt contains live cultures, as indicated on the label) and in capsule form available in health food stores. Take one capsule three times daily.

- Add garlic to your diet, either in its natural form, or in capsule form available from health food stores.

- Take a form of caprylic acid — either Capricin or Caprystatin — and follow the directions on the container as to dosage.

> There is a prescription drug called Nystatin that can be of help to confirmed cases of candidiasis. If you try the yeast-free diet and your symptoms are alleviated but do not completely clear, then you might have had candidiasis for so long that you will require additional treatment in the form of prescription drugs. You should discuss Nystatin with your doctor as it can help you improve at an even faster rate.

CHAPTER 8

Carpal Tunnel Syndrome

Sue-Ann, a patient of mine for several years, is a cheerful, energetic woman who puts in long hours as a legal secretary. I've seen Sue-Ann through various problems ranging from the flu to a sprained ankle and have never heard her complain, but when she came into my office last winter she looked tired and unhappy. "This is killing me," she said, pointing to her wrist. "There's this burning pain that shoots up into my arm and even the shoulder — it's bad enough during the day, but it keeps me awake at night."

Sue-Ann was not surprised to hear she was suffering from carpal tunnel syndrome, a trauma disorder that affects people whose jobs entail making repetitive movements of the hands and wrists. Keyboard operators and carpenters are an example of occupations at risk for carpal tunnel syndrome, with women at higher risk than men.

Typically, Sue-Ann's problem had started out with a tingling sensation in her thumb and forefingers, and, over the next few weeks, had progressed from weakness and numbness of the hand to the burning pain she was now experiencing.

What Is Carpal Tunnel Syndrome?

The problem starts when the ligaments that pass through the wrist — which is known as the carpal tunnel — become inflamed and swell in response to repeated stressful motions. These swollen ligaments press against the median nerve which also runs through the wrist, and the more they press, the greater the discomfort and the pain. Certain conditions such as arthritis, gout, diabetes, pregnancy and thyroid problems can predispose you to developing carpal tunnel syndrome, and it's been suggested that women around menopause are more likely to develop it because hormonal changes may cause fluid build-up and swelling of the wrist.

Do You Have Carpal Tunnel: A Simple Test

There's a simple test you can do yourself to determine if you have carpal tunnel syndrome. Hold out the painful wrist and hand, and, with the fingers of your other hand, tap the wrist where it joins the hand. A tingling shooting down into the hand and fingers indicates you're likely to have carpal tunnel syndrome.

Carpal Tunnel And Surgery

When I examined Sue-Ann's wrist, I showed her the simple technique outlined above to determine if she really had carpal tunnel or if she had simply strained her wrist. When I tapped her wrist, she winced.

"Will I have to have surgery?" she asked.

I assured Sue-Ann that surgery would be a last recourse. While surgery for carpal tunnel syndrome is usually successful, a recent study indicates that two years after surgery, almost one-third of the patients had recurring problems. Natural therapy, on the other hand, is both simple and usually very effective.

First Steps For Carpal Tunnel

I told Sue-Ann that the first thing she must do is rest her wrist to allow the inflammation to subside. I recommended she use a splint to limit movement of the wrist, and that she use heat — either a heating pad or hot bath — at least twice a day. After one week, she could start using her hand again, while still limiting flexion and extension of the wrist.

Fortunately, as a senior legal secretary, Sue-Ann could call on typists from the typing pool, and would not have to use a keyboard until her wrist mended. Once she did, I urged her to take time off at regular intervals to give her wrists a break. Just making a few small circles in the air with her hands would improve circulation and keep her ligaments from irritation.

In the meantime, as she allowed her ligaments to heal through rest, she could complete the healing process through Vitamin B supplementation. Vitamin B^6 strengthens the sheath that surrounds the tendon.

Research has shown that many people who suffer from carpal tunnel syndrome also suffer from a vitamin B^6 deficiency, and Vitamin B^6 supplementation relieved their inflammation and pain. You must be patient, because it takes from six to twelve weeks for the effects to be felt. In addition to Vitamin B^6, I recommended supplements of B^2 and B^{12} to make the treatment more effective. I also recommended folic acid.

Acupuncture For Carpal Tunnel

I told Sue-Ann that, until the natural therapy took effect, she could ease her discomfort and pain with acupuncture treatments. Many of my patients have had enormous success using acupuncture treatments for their carpal tunnel syndrome and many have found permanent relief. If you do decide to try acupuncture, find someone who is highly recommended and well-trained.

Sue-Ann didn't go in for acupuncture treatments (she explained sheepishly that she was terrified of any kind of needles), but she did call me nine weeks later to report that her pain had almost disappeared, and was improving every day. I warned her that the problem might come back if she discontinued Vitamin B supplementation; however, since Vitamin B^6 can be toxic at high levels over long periods of time, I reminded Sue-Ann to switch over to the maintenance dosage.

A Natural Treatment For Carpal Tunnel Syndrome

In addition to your basic daily antioxidant vitamin/mineral supplement, take:

- Vitamin B^6: 300 mg. daily for *no longer than* 3 months; 50–100 mg. daily as a maintenance dosage. Remember that it can take up to three months for the effects of the supplementation to be felt. **Warning:** Vitamin B^6 can be toxic at high levels. Do not take more than the recommended amount.

- Vitamin B^2: 100 mg. daily.

- Vitamin B^{12}: 1000 micrograms daily in tablet form dissolved under the tongue.

- Folic acid: 800 micrograms daily.

Also:

- You may want to use a simple splint — available at a pharmacy — to immobilize the hand and relieve pain until the vitamin B^6 begins to take effect.

- A heating pad or a warm moist compress can help relieve pain.

- If you work at repetitive tasks, stop occasionally and make slow circles with your hands to restore circulation and relieve pressure.

CHAPTER 9 — *Cervical Dysplasia*

There's a great deal of misunderstanding about the Pap test and its results. The Pap smear — a sampling of the cells of the cervix — is the most common screening test for cervical dysplasia, or abnormality of the cells of the cervix, the lowest part of the uterus.

The system that's been in place for years provides five different classifications. Class 1 indicates normal cells and class 5 indicates cancerous cells. But the confusion rises from the classes in between. They indicate some level of abnormality, but not how much, or how serious. A woman who is told she has a "Class 3 Pap smear" is going to be greatly alarmed and wonder about the significance of the result — a significance which not even her doctor may be able to explain.

Elizabeth, who is an editor at a weekly news magazine, came to consult me after being told by her doctor she had an "abnormal" class 3 Pap smear. Her reaction was typical of patients with cervical dysplasia: anxiety, confusion, and a desperate need for information. She came virtually running into my office, sweeping long dark hair off her face with one hand while reaching out to greet me with the other.

"I've been having Pap smears half my life, and always thought they gave you either negative or positive results — that either you had cancer or you didn't. But this gray area, this uncertainty — I can't sleep at night, and I can't concentrate at work. My gynecologist told me he'd schedule another test in a couple of months, but in the meantime I'm going to go crazy, just waiting around."

It's not surprising that Elizabeth was confused and terrified, because there's always been a great deal of confusion regarding the precise significance of different levels of abnormalities, with the interpretation depending on both the laboratory and the physician. In fact, *The Wall Street Journal* recently reported the alarming failure of some laboratories to detect Pap smear abnormalities and report them promptly to the patients.

To eliminate this general confusion, many laboratories are adopting a new system for interpreting Pap smears, called the Bethesda system, which uses uniform terminology and provides clear diagnostic results. But, regardless of which system is used, the Pap smear test is a valuable diagnostic tool, and should be a routine part of every woman's healthcare.

Nutritional Therapy For Cervical Dysplasia

I told Elizabeth she should think of her abnormal Pap result as an alert. If the next test showed progression of her cervical dysplasia to a cancerous level, she would need surgery. But, while waiting for the next test, she would have the opportunity to use nutritional therapy to improve, and eventually cure, her condition.

Many doctors don't realize the effectiveness of nutritional therapy for cervical dysplasia, and merely schedule another test. But a number of patients have used therapy successfully, and have gone from an abnormal test to one that's totally normal. They have reversed the abnormal Pap smear naturally.

Folic acid deficiency is closely linked with the development of cervical cancer, and many patients are very excited when they learn that sometimes, by simply taking folate supplements, any abnormality in a Pap smear will be gone upon retesting. Indeed, folic acid is a sort of miracle supplement for cervical dysplasia. Vitamins A and C can also help reverse cervical dysplasia.

Risk Factors For Cervical Dysplasia

I explained the known risk factors connected with cervical cancer to Elizabeth. Sexual activity at a young age, multiple sexual partners and long-term use of oral contraceptives can all contribute to abnormalities of cervical cells. So can two viruses: the herpes virus and the human papilloma, or wart, virus. And so does smoking.

But there's also strong evidence that nutritional deficiencies play a key role in the development of cancer, and blood tests of cervical cancer patients have shown that at least 67 percent had one or more abnormal vitamin level.

Elizabeth did not smoke, so quitting that was not an issue. And she agreed to take the nutritional supplements recommended for cervical dysplasia. "At least I'll feel I'm doing something positive," she said, "instead of just waiting around for the next test."

I asked Elizabeth to call me with the results of her next Pap smear, which would be scheduled by her gynecologist. I suggested she ask to have it done in the middle of her menstrual cycle, and that she refrain from douching before the test. I also suggested that she ask the lab to use the Bethesda system.

Elizabeth's story had a happy ending. Two months after the first test, she had a second Pap smear, and the results came back absolutely normal, and remained normal the following year.

Many women are unnecessarily frightened by Pap test results: only one in ten precancerous lesions discovered in a Pap smear is likely to develop into cancer if left untreated. If your Pap smear detects an abnormal condition, you can help to normalize it by giving up smoking, and taking nutritional supplements.

The prescription cream Retin A, now used for acne and wrinkles, may have additional health benefits — reversing cervical dysplasia. In a recent study financed by the National Cancer Institute, dysplasia reverted to normal tissue in 43 percent of the cases of women applying Retin A to their cervixes compared to 23 percent of those using a placebo cream. The medication contains a synthetic variation of Vitamin A. Ask your doctor about this.

Nutritional Supplements For Cervical Dysplasia

As I mentioned above, deficiency of folic acid is closely linked to the development of cervical dysplasia. There are reports of women whose cervical dysplasia cleared up after taking folate supplements.

Deficiencies in Vitamins A and B are also linked to cervical dysplasia. In one study, women deficient in Vitamin A were at three times greater risk of severe dysplasia than women with a normal Vitamin A level. Vitamin A and beta-carotene supplements have been reported to clear up cervical dysplasia.

Vitamin C is also important in preventing cervical dysplasia, and women who consume less than 50 percent of the RDA of Vitamin C have ten times the risk of developing dysplasia.

A Natural Treatment For Cervical Dysplasia

- If you smoke, stop. This is important, as smoking is closely linked with the development of dysplasia.

In addition to your daily basic antioxidant vitamin/mineral supplement, take:

- Folic acid: 5 mg. twice a day for three months or until your follow-up Pap smear. (Folic acid comes in 800 microgram tablets; you need to take about 9 a day and you can take them all at one time.) Also increase your consumption of foods rich in folic acid, including raw, deep-green leafy vegetables such as spinach, beet greens, kale, turnip greens, broccoli, asparagus, as well as endive, liver, wheat germ and lima beans.

- Vitamin A: 60,000 I.U. daily for two months; then 25,000 I.U. daily or until follow-up Pap smear. Alternatively, take 25,000 I.U. of beta-carotene daily. Also increase your consumption of foods rich in vitamin A, including carrots, squash, sweet potatoes, dark leafy vegetables and broccoli.

- Vitamin C: 1000 mg. daily.

Surgery For Cervical Dysplasia

If subsequent testing indicates that you do require surgery, the standard treatment is a cone biopsy which takes a cone-shaped biopsy of the cervix. The procedure must be done in an operating room under general or spinal anesthesia. But there is a new treatment called LEEP, or Loop Electrosurgical Excision Procedure, which was developed in Britain and is becoming increasingly available in this country.

LEEP has many advantages over cone biopsy in that it requires only local anesthesia, is fast, causes no post-op pain or discomfort and no opportunity for infection following the procedure. Of course, your doctor is the best judge of what procedure is appropriate for your condition but, if indicated, LEEP could simplify your treatment.

CHAPTER 10

Congestive Heart Failure

Jennie, who's been a patient of mine for several years, called me a year ago to tell me how worried she was about her mother Sara, who was suffering from congestive heart failure. "She's seen a heart specialist, and is taking regular medication, but she's tired all the time — she gets breathless just crossing the room."

I told Jennie that I would have to see her mother before I could determine how she could be helped. I explained that you cannot cure congestive heart failure through natural therapies, but you can use them in addition to standard medications to further alleviate the symptoms.

What Is Congestive Heart Failure?

Congestive heart failure is caused when the pumping action of the heart is impaired, usually as a result of a serious disease. High blood pressure, heart valve disease, heart attack, emphysema, congenital heart disease, and atherosclerosis (hardening of the arteries) can all result in congestive heart failure.

As the heart becomes less and less efficient at pumping blood, fluid accumulates in the veins that carry the blood from the lungs, and the lungs become swollen and congested. The legs may also become swollen with fluid, and the patient may also become breathless, particularly after mild exercise, or may find it difficult to breathe when lying down. Congestive heart failure can also cause chest pains, appetite loss, frequent urination, particularly at night, and mental confusion.

Sara came to see me two weeks after her daughter called. She was a retired schoolteacher in her mid-sixties, but her slow movements and her hesitant way of speaking made her seem frail and much older. She was sad and depressed, not so much because of her illness as for the fact that it would force her to cancel her long-standing plans. She and two of her friends had been saving to spend the winter together in Florida — they'd signed a lease on a Miami condominium — and now Sara was afraid she'd have to drop out.

Sara told me that the first symptoms she had experienced were breathlessness and fatigue. These are the first symptoms experienced by most patients, and if you have these symptoms you should see a doctor right away, because anyone with congestive heart failure needs to be under the care of a physician.

"But it's been getting worse recently" Sara told me. "Now I'm having trouble sleeping at night — soon as I lie down I find it difficult to breathe — and so of course I'm exhausted the next day. And the medications don't really seem to help."

Sara was taking digitalis, to stimulate her heart, and diuretics, to rid her body of excess fluids. Some patients with congestive heart failure are also given a drug called Procardia. I told Sara, as I've told my other patients with congestive heart failure, that it was essential to continue taking the medications prescribed by their physicians. But I also told Sara that natural therapy could help ease her symptoms, as it has for many of my patients.

The first thing I noticed, when Sara came back to see me a month later, was that she walked with greater energy and confidence, and that she had taken the trouble to put on some makeup. I asked her if she felt better, and she nodded.

"I've been sleeping really well at night," she explained, "and it makes all the difference. In fact, I hardly ever feel short of breath anymore. I give Co-enzyme Q-10 the credit — I started feeling better a week or so after I started taking it. And I've been eating the fruits and vegetables you suggested, And taking the other supplements, of course."

Sara was typical of many of my patients in finding relief from the symptoms of congestive heart failure. Her improvement was such that her heart specialist gave her permission to join her friends in Florida for the winter, where she continued to improve.

Many other patients with congestive heart failure have also shown a remarkable improvement of symptoms when using natural therapy in conjunction with their prescribed medications.

You Must Consult A Doctor

If you suspect you may have congestive heart failure, you should be under the care of your regular physician. The following recommendations are meant to supplement your own doctor's prescriptions and recommended treatment.

Improve Your Nutritional Status

A healthy diet is of paramount importance to women with a heart problem. Eat a balanced diet as described in A HEALTHY WOMAN'S DAILY ROUTINE, page 19. In addition, to discourage the retention of fluid in the system, cut down on your salt intake. And eat at least 5 one-half cup helpings of fruits and vegetables rich in beta-carotene, as described below.

Nutritional Supplements For Congestive Heart Failure

Coenzyme Q-10, also known as ubiquinone, is enormously helpful to people with heart disease and I recommend to all of my patients with symptoms of heart disease that they add it to their daily regime. It plays a role in fat and energy metabolism, and helps to prevent the accumulation of fatty acids in the heart.

You may have heard that the FDA claims Co Q-10 has no benefits, and indeed tried to ban it at one time, but consumers have fought to keep it in the stores because it's been so helpful. My own patients report improvement of their symptoms within one to three weeks of taking Co Q-10.

Carnitine is another nutritional supplement that strengthens the heart by burning fatty acids. Carnitine also helps in lowering total cholesterol and triglyceride levels and prevents irregular heartbeat. It improves the heart's overall tolerance for exercise. Carnitine is naturally produced by the body, but production decreases as people age. I advise my patients with congestive heart failure to take DL-carnitine daily.

Another supplement that can provide relief is beta-carotene, which reduces symptoms significantly, and reduces the risk of strokes, heart attacks and sudden cardiac death. Beta-carotene is especially effective when taken in the fruits and vegetables which are its primary sources.

I recommend that my patients with congestive heart failure consume at least five half-cup servings of yellow/orange fruits and vegetables such as cantaloupe, apricots, peaches, carrots and sweet potatoes, and dark-green leafy vegetables such as broccoli, kale, spinach and arugula. To make sure that they have a sufficient amount of beta-carotene, I also tell my patients to take a supplement daily.

Magnesium is also essential to the proper functions of the heart. It is used to control the irregular heartbeats that patients with congestive heart failure are prone to, in the form of premature ventricular contractions. As many as 20 percent of patients with congestive heart failure have magnesium deficiencies. I recommend daily supplements to my heart patients.

Vitamin E has also been linked to the health of the heart, and low levels of vitamin E increase the risk of various heart problems. Indeed, one World Health Organization study found low levels of vitamin E to be a major risk factor for death from heart disease.

Exercise and Your Heart

Exercise is important for strengthening the heart, and making it more resistant to failure. But people with heart disease can have particular concerns when it comes to exercise. I don't recommend that you embark on an exercise program without consulting your doctor. A physician will be able to recommend an exercise program that will be safe and manageable for your condition.

A Natural Treatment For Congestive Heart Failure

If you have congestive heart failure, you should be under the regular care of a physician. The following suggestions are meant to complement your doctor's recommendations.

In addition to your basic daily antioxidant vitamin/mineral supplement, take:

- Coenzyme Q-10: 30 to 60 mg. three times a day.
- DL-carnitine: 250 mg. three times a day.
- Beta-carotene: five half-cup servings of fruits and vegetables daily such as yellow/orange fruits and vegetables, including carrots, sweet potatoes, apricots, peaches and cantaloupes and dark-green leafy vegetables such as broccoli, spinach, kale and arugula. Alternatively, you can take take beta-carotene supplements in the amount of 25,000 mg. daily.
- Magnesium: 250 mg. twice daily.
- Vitamin E: 400 I.U. daily.
- Exercise: Discuss with your doctor.

CHAPTER 11

Constipation

At the end of a routine visit not long ago, a woman patient of mine who is in good health mentioned that she had recently been troubled by constipation. Her diet hadn't changed, nor had any of her health habits, but the constipation was becoming a real problem and she couldn't figure out what was causing it. This patient, at the age of 49, was in perimenopause — she was probably a year or two away from actual menopause but she was beginning to notice symptoms common to this stage of a woman's life.

Constipation can be one of these symptoms. Just as the hormonal changes of pregnancy can cause constipation, so the hormonal fluctuations of menopause can result in constipation. This patient had never experienced constipation, had no idea that it could be related in any way to menopause, and was truly confused about what was causing it and how to cope with it.

Generally speaking, people tend to average one bowel movement a day. But people vary greatly from one another in the frequency of their bowel movements, so that one person may have one or more stools a day, whereas the next person will only have one every other day. In my years of practice, I've found that many more people think of themselves as constipated than truly are. You may be constipated if the pattern of your bowel movements has changed and has become irregular or infrequent, and if your stools are hard, small, and difficult to pass.

I certainly believe that more frequent bowel movements are better, because it's healthier to eliminate the waste from your bowel as soon as possible, so as to avoid potential problems. That does not mean that I advocate the use of laxatives to promote more frequent or regular stools. On the contrary. Laxatives are very helpful on occasion, but their indiscriminate use can actually encourage constipation by creating a "lazy" bowel. Moreover, frequent use of laxatives can deplete your body of the mineral potassium which is crucial for proper heart functioning.

Also, since constipation is a symptom and not a disease, the regular use of laxatives camouflages the symptom without curing the cause. If you must use a laxative on occasion, try the "natural" or "vegetable" laxatives — the ones made from crushed psyllium seed. They are not addictive and are usually effective.

> If you become constipated very suddenly, have stomach pain and cramps, and can't even pass gas, you may have developed an obstruction that requires immediate medical attention.

Constipation: A Simple Cause

For most people, constipation is a result of bad habits and poor diet. Many women develop constipation simply because they don't take time out for a bowel movement, even when they feel the urge to do so. One young mother of two told me that she used to be as regular as clockwork, but when the children started going to school, things just got too hectic in the morning. "I've got to get dressed for work, and make sure the kids get dressed for school, and get breakfast on the table. . .there's just no time for anything else."

Another patient of mine, an executive whose job takes her frequently out of town, told me that traveling really throws her off her routine. "Sometimes I'll go two or three days without a bowel movement," she said, "and then I get to the point where I must use a laxative."

I tell my patients that ignoring the urge to move their bowels is a sure way to get constipated. A regular routine, sufficient fiber in the diet, enough liquids to drink, and a moderate amount of exercise will promote regular bowel movements, and will prevent constipation and related problems.

Laxative Addiction

Occasionally I see a patient who has used laxatives for so long that's she's become addicted to them and cannot move her bowels without them. In this case, I recommend that you take your laxative (one containing either cascara or senna) at night, just before bed. Use the toilet in the morning at the same time each day.

After one week of this routine, decrease the laxative amount by half (take just enough to insure that you will have a bowel movement the next day). Each week, decrease the laxative dosage by half until you have weaned yourself from the medication entirely.

Follow A Regular Routine

Set aside a few minutes each day, preferably after breakfast, to sit on the toilet — even if you don't feel an urge — and try to have a bowel movement. I don't mean you should strain, because that causes hemorrhoids, but just give your system a chance to work. To help things along, a hot drink followed by a cold drink can stimulate bowel contractions. It's best if you can use the toilet at the same time each day.

Try to follow the same routine whether you are at home, at work, or traveling. By following a regular routine, you can actually "train" your bowels to move at the same time each day.

The Importance Of Regular Exercise

Regular exercise is another habit that will help to prevent constipation. When you exercise, you stimulate your system to work more efficiently, and to move food faster through your bowels. In addition, exercise is essential to your overall good health. Just a twenty minute walk four or five times a week will make a big difference.

Add Fiber To Your Diet

Another major cause of constipation is a lack of enough fiber in the diet. This is easily remedied by adding fresh fruits, grains and vegetables to your diet: good for your overall health. I recommend fruit for breakfast, a fruit snack in the afternoon and one in the evening, and of course fresh vegetables at dinner.

If fresh fruits and vegetables are not sufficient, adding some bran to the diet may be helpful. I recommend coarse miller's bran, which you can take with fruit, juice, cereal or yogurt. For some people, one spoonful of bran is sufficient, while others require up to half a cup. You can experiment until you find the amount that's right for you.

Some people discover that they don't tolerate any amount of bran, because it makes them feel gassy. A reaction that involves a lot of gas and bloating after taking bran could mean that you have celiac disease, also known as sprue. Celiac disease is a sensitivity to gluten, the protein found in wheat and other grains. If you think you have celiac disease, discuss it with your doctor.

An alternative to bran is psyllium powder, available at many drug stores and health food stores. Be sure to follow the instructions on the label and drink enough water — without it, the psyllium powder won't be effective, and can actually cause a bowel obstruction.

Med Alert!

Sometimes medications can cause constipation. Antacids containing aluminum or calcium, antihistamines, anti-Parkinsonism drugs, calcium supplements, diuretics, narcotics, phenothiazines, sedatives and tricyclic antidepressants can all contribute to constipation. If you suspect that a medication may be the cause of your constipation, consult with your doctor.

Water: The Secret Ingredient

Many people develop constipation simply because *they don't drink enough water.* This happened to some of my patients who took my advice to cut back on diet sodas and caffeinated drinks, but failed to otherwise increase their liquid intake!

You should drink between four and six glasses of water a day. A good way to remember is to keep a bottle of club soda or mineral water within easy reach during the day, and drink from it at regular intervals.

Some of my patients have told me that they keep six or eight pennies in one pocket and each time they drink a glass of water, they move a penny to another pocket. The goal is to have the original pocket empty at the end of the day.

Aloe Vera Capsules

Some of my patients have found aloe vera gel caps to be effective in encouraging a bowel movement. You can buy aloe vera gel caps in your health food store.

A Natural Treatment For Constipation

- Be sure you're getting adequate fiber in your diet. Eat plenty of fresh fruits and vegetables as well as whole grain cereals.
- Add bran to your diet. I recommend coarse miller's bran. Begin with one tablespoon in the morning and gradually increase by a tablespoon every several days until you achieve the desired result. You can mix it in juice or yogurt or sprinkle it on cereal. If the bran causes too much gas and bloating (it usually does

cause some) cut down on the amount or try:

- Psyllium fiber stool bulking agent. Follow the directions on the package and **be sure to drink adequate amounts of water**. Usually you take one teaspoon in a glass of water and increase to two teaspoons a day if necessary.

- Try aloe vera gel capsules which are a natural stimulant to move the bowels. Follow the directions on the package. They're available in natural food stores.

- Drink plenty of fluids: *four to six glasses of water each day.*

- Develop healthy bowel habits. Give yourself time to use the toilet at least once each day, at the same time each day, usually after breakfast. Drink something hot followed by something cold and then relax on the toilet. Don't strain. Be sure to go whenever you feel the urge.

- If you must use a laxative, do so only occasionally and try to stick with the "natural" or "vegetable" laxatives made from concentrated psyllium seeds.

CHAPTER 12

Cystitis

If your pattern of urination changes suddenly, and you feel a frequent urge to urinate, accompanied by pain or a burning sensation, you may have cystitis.

Cystitis is a bladder infection that will affect almost half the women in the country at some point in their lives, while 20 percent of all women are prone to chronic infections of cystitis.

The bacteria that cause cystitis travel to the bladder through the urethra. Women suffer from cystitis much more frequently than men because of their basic anatomy: the proximity of the urethra to the anus makes it easily accessible to fecal bacteria. The bacteria may also be transmitted on your unwashed hands or the hands and genitals of a sexual partner. And then there are women who are predisposed to cystitis through an anatomical condition.

Causes Of Cystitis

While fecal bacteria are the most frequent cause of female cystitis, vigorous and frequent intercourse can also create a climate that promotes cystitis: in fact, the infection has sometimes been called "honeymoon cystitis."

Infrequent urination is another cause of bladder cystitis because, the longer you hold the urine in your bladder, the more opportunity any bacteria present have to duplicate. When you consider that the bacteria double every twenty minutes, you realize that even short delays can cause you a real problem. Recent studies have shown that women who ignore the urge to urinate are far more likely to develop a bladder infection than women who urinate as soon as they feel the urge.

Complications Of Cystitis

Once the infection is in your system, it can spread to adjacent organs. If, in addition to a painful and burning sensation when you urinate, you also experience a fever, and a low back pain, or blood in your urine, you may have developed a kidney infection. Cystitis, as well as kidney infections, are treated with antibiotics prescribed by your doctor.

The bad news is that repeated use of antibiotics can actually increase your potential for future infection, because antibiotics kill off the "good" bacteria along with the bad. The good news is that you can use some very effective natural treatments to help prevent future infections.

Good Hygiene Is Essential

Scrupulous hygiene is the best way of preventing cystitis.

- Make sure your hands are clean before you go to the toilet, (yes, it's a good idea to wash your hands before as well as after!) and wipe from front to back to avoid spreading fecal matter from the anus to the genital area and the urethra.
- Keep your genital area clean and dry, avoid tight, clinging clothes, and wear cotton panties.
- Feminine hygiene sprays, douches and bubble baths which may spread infection are also best avoided.

A Simple Prevention For Cystitis

Since frequent emptying of the bladder flushes it clean of bacteria, try to void frequently, or whenever you feel the urge. The minute that it takes will save you a lot of time, trouble and discomfort later. Many women who suffer from frequent bouts of cystitis are very busy and simply avoid using the toilet. They may go for hours and hours between "stops." This bad habit encourages the growth of harmful bacteria and frequent bouts of cystitis.

Drink Lots Of Water

In order to void frequently and flush out your system, you need to drink plentiful amounts of fluids, particularly water. I tell my patients they should drink at least six eight-ounce glasses of water daily. Try the trick of putting eight pennies in your right pocket, moving one to your left pocket each time you drink a glass of water. At the end of the day you want all your pennies in the left pocket!

Sip Before Sex

To decrease the odds of infection developing from intercourse, drink fluids before intercourse, and void your bladder soon afterward. This will flush out your urethra and prevent infection.

In addition, wash the genital area shortly after intercourse.

The Cranberry Cure

At one time, doctors thought the use of cranberry juice for urinary tract problems was based on nothing more substantial than an old wives' tale. Later, some doctors thought that cranberry juice was beneficial because it helped to "acidify" the urine. Now we know that cranberry juice is effective because it actually prevents bacteria from adhering to the lining of the urethra and the bladder.

Since the cranberry juice sold at grocery stores is very high in sugar, I recommend that you take cranberry concentrate, or cranberry concentrate capsules, both of which are available at your health food store.

Nutritional Supplements For Cystitis

I tell my patients who suffer from cystitis to take buffered vitamin C to help fight the infection, as well as bioflavonoids, zinc, and vitamin A which helps to acidify the urine.

Another Possible Cause. . .

If you've been treated with antibiotics for a bladder and kidney infection and continue experiencing frequent and painful urination after the antibiotic treatment is finished, you may be suffering from a yeast overgrowth known as Candidiasis, which often develops when the "good" bacteria which control yeast are killed off along with the bad bacteria. If you've had frequent bladder infections, or if you're suffering complications after antibiotic treatment, I recommend you go on a yeast-cleansing program for three months. Refer to **Candidiasis**, page 115.

A Natural Treatment For Cystitis

For Prevention:

- Practice good personal hygiene: wipe from front to back after having a bowel movement and keep the vaginal area clean and dry.
- Avoid feminine hygiene sprays, douches, and bubble baths.
- Avoid tight clothing and wear cotton panties.
- Urinate frequently, as soon as you feel the urge. Never hold your urine.
- Drink lots of fluids: try to consume at least 6 eight-ounce glasses of water daily. Avoid citrus juices for the duration of any infection.
- Drink fluids before intercourse and void soon afterward.

For Treatment:

- Drink cranberry juice (try the low-calorie kind) or, better still, try cranberry extract capsules. Take one capsule three times a day with an eight-ounce glass of water.

In addition to your daily basic antioxidant vitamin/ mineral supplement, take:

- Vitamin C: 500 mg. every 2 hours for the duration of the infection and cut down to

1000 to 1,500 mg. daily for a maintenance dose once the infection has cleared.

- Bioflavonoids: one gram daily.
- Vitamin A: 25,000 I.U. daily during the infection.
- Zinc: 30 mg. daily.

Also:

- If bladder infections are persistent, try a yeast-cleansing diet by avoiding foods containing yeast, including bread, cheese, mushrooms, vinegar, soy sauce, fermented foods, alcohol, olives, pickles, etc. In addition, take acidophilus supplements: one capsule three times daily. For more information on yeast, see CANDIDIASIS, page 115.

If you have regular bladder infections, you should have a urologic exam and a specialized X-ray to see if there's any abnormality of the urethra.

CHAPTER 13 — *Depression*

Depression is one of our most misunderstood disorders, and many people think it's synonymous with disappointment and sadness. They complain about the depressing weather, or of feeling depressed during the holidays, and don't realize that true depression is a painful and disabling disorder that requires medical attention.

Such was the case with Denise, a woman in her early forties who had consulted me a year earlier about a minor skin disorder. I remembered her as an attractive, energetic woman with an infectious smile, and I was concerned when she walked into my office: she looked thin and listless, dimmed in some way, as though someone had wiped both coloring and expression from her face.

"There's nothing really wrong with me," was the first thing she said. "My husband insisted that

I come to see you, but there's nothing anyone can do. I'm just feeling depressed."

As I talked to Denise to diagnose the extent of her depression, I had the impression that she seemed indifferent, as though she were talking about a stranger she didn't know very well. She had been depressed about for three months, she said. She didn't know what had brought it on. Nothing, or maybe everything.

She and her husband were thrilled when she got pregnant last spring — their daughter was going off to college in the fall, and it would be wonderful to have another child around the house — but she had miscarried in her third month. The boutique she had managed had gone out of business, and she had been unable to get another job — they were hiring younger, prettier women, she said. And the family dog — her dog, really — had died of old age.

She was always tired, Denise said. She would sleep for a few hours at night, but she always seemed to wake up at three or four in the morning, and she wouldn't go back to sleep until after her husband had left for work. I gathered she often skipped meals, and that some days she didn't even bother getting dressed. Her family and some of her friends her told her to "snap out" of it, but she didn't have the energy.

"I just feel so tired all the time," said Denise, "and sort of empty and gray, if you know what I mean." I diagnosed Denise as suffering from clinical depression.

Depression Versus Sadness

It's normal for people who've lost a job or a loved one — even a pet — to suffer from overwhelming sadness, but people who lose their ability to function on an everyday basis are suffering from depression and need medical help.

The American Psychiatric Association has described clinical depression as "the loss of interest or pleasure in all or almost all usual activities and pastimes." You don't "snap out" of clinical depression, and well-meaning people who urge their relatives to do so are only making things worse, by adding feelings of worthlessness and guilt to the patient's already precarious state.

The True Toll Of Depression

I told Denise that depression requires medical treatment and attention, and that, in one large study conducted by the RAND Corporation and UCLA, depression was shown to be more disabling than serious disorders such as arthritis, ulcers, diabetes, or high blood pressure. Only arthritis was more painful, and only advanced heart disease caused the patient to spend more days in bed.

Furthermore, we now know that depression affects both physical health and mortality rates. For instance, one study of 330 men with HIV — the virus that causes AIDS — showed that, within three years after diagnosis, those who were depressed died at twice the rate of those without depression. Fortunately, depression, which is often due to a biochemical reaction, can be successively treated with drugs, psychotherapy, or both.

Depression And Menopause

Some women find that the changing levels of the hormones estrogen and progesterone at the time of menopause have a powerful effect on their moods — to the point where they begin to feel depressed for the first time in their lives. At the same time, they may be experiencing insomnia, hot flashes, water retention, fatigue, tingling and numbness in the hands and feet.

Some women become so concerned about these other symptoms and so confused about what's related to menopause and what's not, they are even more vulnerable to depression. If you think that menopause may be contributing to your depression, see the chapter on **Menopause**, page 265, for suggestions on natural treatments that will alleviate your symptoms.

Involve An Expert

As I expected, Denise seemed encouraged to realize she was suffering from a real — and treatable — disorder, and not an imaginary disease of her own creation. I urged Denise to see a mental health specialist for treatment. It's important to consult someone knowledgeable about severe depression because, if a prescription is written by a primary care physician who lacks the experience to prescribe the right medication and dose, the treatment will not work.

The Natural Approach

While treatment by a mental health specialist is essential for someone with a severe depression, natural therapy can help to make that treatment more effective, and I encouraged Denise to try the natural therapy guidelines I discuss below. I did not see Denise for several months, but when she came to my office I was glad to see that she seemed more like her old self.

"It took me a while to respond to the antidepressants," she told me. "And then I realized that I'd really let myself get run down. And it's not really fair to my family, is it? So I've been eating well and taking Vitamin C and a Vitamin B complex, as you recommended. Also, I'm back into my exercise routine. I started out by walking for half an hour each day and now I'm back to working out at my regular gym. And I've been going on a lot of job interviews, and I'm pretty sure I've got something lined up at a department store. I'm to go back for a third interview next week."

Causes Of Depression

Depression can be brought on by a variety of things. People with a family history of depression are more likely to experience it. Chronic diseases and alcoholism can cause depression, and so can infectious diseases such as hepatitis, mononucleosis, and tuberculosis. Hormonal fluctuations can set it off, as in the case of women suffering postpartum depression, or women who experience it before their menstrual cycle.

Hidden food allergies can also cause various mental symptoms, including depression, and one study found that 85 percent of a group of depressed adults and children were allergic. Another interesting study found that 33 percent of depressed patients had food allergies, compared to only 2 percent in a control group of schizophrenics.

People with low blood sugar or hypoglycemia often suffer from a constant mild depression when their irregular eating habits cause rapid fluctuations of blood sugar levels.

Depression And SAD

And then there is the depression that affects people in northern climates in the winter, when light is reduced. It's called Seasonal Affective Disorder (SAD) and it usually starts with the shorter days in autumn, peaks in January, and improves once the days start getting longer.

It's been suggested that people who suffer from the "holiday blues," particularly at Christmastime, are really suffering from SAD. People who suffer from SAD are four times more likely to be women, and in particular women whose jobs don't take them outdoors.

We don't know exactly what causes SAD, but we do know that when light enters the retina of our eyes, electrical impulses send messages to the hypothalamus, which in turn relays chemical and electrical messages to the brain and other parts of the body. People who are blind react the same way as people with vision, which explains how the blind remain synchronized to dark and light rhythms.

Ellen, a young woman in her mid-twenties with two small children at home, had symptoms typical of a SAD patient. She complained of a lack of energy and an urge to oversleep and overeat starchy foods, which had caused her to gain weight. In addition, she felt anxious much of the time, and, though in love with her husband, had lost most of her interest in sex.

Fortunately, Ellen responded quickly to a regimen of supplements of melatonin, a hormone that promotes sleepiness when it grows dark, taken in conjunction with light therapy, which is simply a daily exposure to bright fluorescent light.

Whatever the cause or severity of depression, patients can be helped by natural therapy as an adjunct to their regular treatment, and mild cases of depression can even be headed off by the timely use of natural therapy. Outlined below are the steps you should follow if you (or someone close to you) are suffering from depression.

Do You Need Professional Help?

There are a number of warning signals that flash the need for consultation with a mental specialist. Seek professional help if at least four of these symptoms are present for at least two weeks:

- Altered sleeping habits, such as insomnia, or waking at 4 am.
- Altered eating habits, whether loss of appetite, or weight loss or gain.
- Hyperactivity or underactivity.
- Loss of usual interests.
- Lethargy.
- Feelings of worthlessness and guilt.
- Inability to concentrate.
- Suicidal thoughts or attempted suicide.
- Overwhelming feelings of anxiety, sadness, and emptiness.

When You Need Help. . .

For a referral to a professional in your area, contact the National Mental Health Association, 1021 Prince Street, Alexandria, VA 22314, phone number (703) 684-7722.

Nutrition And Depression

People who are depressed tend to eat erratically, and their inadequate nutrition, in turn, aggravates their depression. Deficiencies of vitamin C and the B complex are frequent in people who suffer from depression. Follow the guidelines in A HEALTHY WOMAN'S DAILY ROUTINE, Page 19, to prevent nutritional problems that can have a direct effect on your state of mind.

Blood Sugar And Depression

I've seen a number of patients who think they might be suffering from depression but instead are victims of low blood sugar. Irregular eating habits, resulting in rapid fluctuations of blood sugar levels, can cause mood swings and symptoms that are typical of depression. Many of these people eat too many sweets — they sometimes refer to themselves as "sugar addicts."

If you believe your depression is the result of low blood sugar, or hypoglycemia, you can stabilize your blood sugar levels by eating regular meals at regular times, by eating protein at both lunch and dinner, and eliminating sugar, caffeine and simple carbohydrates from your diet. In addition, the mineral chromium can be very helpful in stabilizing blood sugar. See HYPOGLYCEMIA, page 243, for detailed information on coping with low blood sugar.

Depression And Food Allergies

If you suffer from hay fever, dust allergies, or allergies to pets, you may also have hidden food allergies that contribute to your depression. One study found that the incidence of allergy was about 33 percent in a group of depressed patients compared with only 2 percent in a control group of schizophrenics. Another study found that 85 percent of a group of depressed children and adults was allergic. It's my experience that wheat is the most common cause of depression among people who are allergic to it.

Exercise And Depression

Exercise can be extremely effective in treating depression.

Most people who are depressed are not physically fit. Exercise will improve their physical condition, and — because the mind and body are so closely bound — their mental one as well. Do as much exercise as you can. You can start with a short walk each day, and work up to a brisk three mile walk; or you can use your stationary bike or work out at your gym.

One woman patient who was being treated for depression found that when she started walking regularly with a friend, it had a dramatic effect on her mood and she credits the exercise with being the factor that really pulled her through the worst of her depression. (It doesn't hurt to do something — any activity — with a friend on a regular basis. It's a guaranteed boost for energy and spirits.)

I recommend exercise to all patients suffering from depression, whether they suffer from SAD, mild depression, or severe depression, and are being treated with psychotherapy and drugs.

Simple Treatments For SAD

If you have Seasonal Affective Disorder, daily exposure to bright fluorescent light is the treatment of choice. This "light therapy," as it's known, requires that you sit in front of a light box that contains full-spectrum fluorescent lights at eye level. In the course of the treatment, you can read, do your nails, or just do nothing, but you must keep your eyes open and near the light source. The light should be about 2,500 lux, as compared to a well-lit room, which is 500 to 750 lux. I recommend you talk to a specialist before starting treatment. Sources for SAD specialists and light boxes are given below.

In addition to the light treatment, try supplements of melatonin, a hormone available at your health food store that can help to regulate your sleeping cycle and combat SAD.

Take a walk at lunchtime to get more exposure to daylight.

Take a winter vacation in a sunny place.

Nutritional Supplements For Depression

Two amino acids have been extremely helpful to some people with depression. Tyrosine, which is often decreased in depressed patients, promotes the synthesis of the neurotransmitter norepinephrine, which helps to promote positive moods, energy and drive. Depressed patients who took a tyrosine supplement reported improved sleeping patterns, mood, libido, and physiological and psychological patterns within the week.

The other amino acid is D-phenylalanine, which is converted into tyrosine by the liver and is also involved in the metabolism of epinephrine, which promotes energy and drive.

Herbal Update. . .

Some recent research has pointed to St. John's wort, a common herb and dietary supplement, as a possible help in relieving depression. In a study reported in <u>The British Medical Journal</u>, more subjects reported an improvement in their depression as a result of St. John's wort than from prescription antidepressants like Elavil, Tofranil and Norpramin. We don't yet know if St. John's wort works for severe depression and whether there are serious side effects over the long term. You should never discontinue use of a prescription medication without consulting your doctor, but you might also investigate the use of St. John's Wort in your battle with depression.

Read To Fight Depression

Reading is another approach you can use to fight depression. In an interesting study, forty-five women and men suffering from mild to moderate depression were given two self-help books: *Feeling Good: The New Mood Therapy* by David D. Burns, and *Control Your Depression*, by Peter Lewisohn. They were asked to read the one of their choosing within four weeks.

At the end of the study, two-thirds of the readers reported significant improvement, compared to a 20 percent improvement reported by the comparison group. Just as important, a follow-up of the readers six months later showed that the improvements were sustained. If you feel reluctant about consulting a psychotherapist, you could start out by reading a self-help book.

A Natural Treatment For Depression

- Many cases of depression require outside help. See the list of signals in this chapter that indicate whether you should be seen by a professional specializing in depression. If necessary, get in touch with an appropriate specialist through the National Mental Health Association (address on page 166) or a referral from your family physician.

- Low blood sugar, or hypoglycemia, is a common cause of depression. For information on the connection between depression and low blood sugar and information on how to use diet and supplements to control low blood sugar, see HYPOGLYCEMIA, page 243.

- Food allergies can cause depression. Avoid allergenic foods. Consult with a doctor who specializes in nutritional medicine for help with this.

In addition to your daily basic antioxidant vitamin/mineral, take:

- Melatonin: 2 mg. at bedtime during the dark months. (I've found that the sublingual tablets — which dissolve under your tongue — are the most effective.)
- Amino acid tyrosine: 500 mg. one or two capsules three times daily.
- Amino acid D-phenylalanine: 500 mg. one or two capsules three times daily.

Also:

- Some cases of depression are caused by Seasonal Affective Disorder (SAD). Light treatment can be extremely helpful for people who suffer from SAD. You can find someone experienced with SAD in your area by contacting the Society for Light Treatment and Biological Rhythms, P.O. Box 478, Wilsonville, OR 97070. Sources for light boxes include: The Sunbox Company (301) 869-5980; Apollo Light Systems, Inc. (801) 226-2370; and Hughes Lighting Technologies (973) 663-1214.

Other tips for people with SAD include:

- Avoid sugar and caffeine which exacerbate depression.
- Take a walk at lunch.
- Take a winter vacation in a sunny place.

- Exercise has been proven to help fight depression. I suggest a half-hour of brisk walking at least five days a week as being the simplest, most readily available form of exercise. Other forms of exercise are just as effective, such as biking, swimming, aerobics classes, etc.

- Avoid sleeping too much as sleeping exacerbates depression.

- Read *Feeling Good: The New Mood Therapy* by David D. Burns and *Control Your Depression* by Peter Lewisohn, both recommended as having proved helpful for many depressed people.

CHAPTER 14 —— *Diverticular Disease*

Diverticulosis used to be a rare disease. Indeed, in many parts of the world it's virtually nonexistent. But in the United States, where our diet contains so many refined foods lacking in fiber, more than half the people over the age of 60 have the condition, often without knowing it.

Diverticulosis is a condition of the colon which occurs when little sacs, or pockets — somewhat like little balloons — develop on the outer walls of the colon from the pressure of hard, dry, and difficult stools.

The symptoms of diverticulosis are gas, chronic constipation which alternates with diarrhea, and sometimes pain in the lower left side of the abdomen. But some people have no symptoms at all, and have no idea there's anything wrong until they progress to the second stage of the disease —

diverticulitis — when fecal matter gets trapped in one of the small sacs, and becomes infected.

Heidi, one of my patients with diverticulitis, came in to see me with her twin sister, Teresa, in tow, obviously in need of moral support. The sisters were in their late sixties, short, round, with round and genial faces. But right then they were both terrified.

"I'm having terrible stomach cramps," said Heidi.

"She has a fever, too," said Teresa.

"And I'm bleeding from the rectum," Heidi whispered.

Heidi and her sister thought she had cancer, and they were immensely relieved when tests revealed that she had diverticulitis. I prescribed antibiotics and asked her to come back in two weeks for a follow-up visit.

> If you have severe cramps or rectal bleeding, you should see your physician right away. Diverticulitis can usually be treated at home with antibiotics, but if it's not treated promptly there may be serious complications requiring surgery to remove the infected segment of the colon. In fact, many physicians recommend surgery after the second bout with diverticulitis.

Fiber, The Simple Cure

When Heidi came back to see me, together with Teresa, we talked about diverticulitis and diverticulosis: her bout with the former (characterized by infection) had passed, but her problem with the latter could be chronic unless she made some modifications in her lifestyle.

The main area of concern was her diet, which I gathered consisted mainly of pasta, meat and potatoes . . . and the occasional dessert. No, she admitted, she seldom ate fresh fruit, salads, or vegetables. Yes, she said, she had always been somewhat constipated and gassy, but she thought it ran in the family, because her sister had much the same trouble.

I told Heidi that her problem was her diet: too much refined food lacking in fiber. To prevent another attack of diverticulitis it was essential that she add fiber to her diet.

I explained to Heidi and Teresa that diverticulitis was an advanced stage of diverticulosis. People who eat high fiber diets all their life never develop diverticulosis. Once it develops, however, you can't get rid of it by eating a high fiber diet — the only way to get rid of the little sacs, once they develop, is through surgery, but you can prevent further complications by eating a high fiber diet. According to various studies, increased fiber can prevent surgical treatment in about 90 percent of patients.

"Is there a chance that I have diverticulosis too?" asked Teresa.

I told her that if she had followed the same diet as her sister, it was highly likely that she did have diverticulosis, even if she was free of symptoms. But I assured her that she, too, could avoid complications if she changed her diet and started taking fiber supplements. In fact, anyone with diverticular disease, whether or not they've had previous complications, can remain symptom-free by following natural therapy.

Improve Your Nutritional Status

Since diverticular disease is caused by a diet of refined foods lacking in fiber, the first thing you must do is change your eating habits. Eat lots of fruits and vegetables, whole grains, and cereals. Eat fruit instead of pastry for a mid-morning or afternoon snack. Avoid processed, refined foods. Instead of white rice, for instance, eat brown rice, richer in fiber and nutrients.

Take A Fiber Supplement

You can add fiber to your diet by taking bran or psyllium powder supplements. Psyllium, which is easier to tolerate, is available over-the-counter in pharmacies, or in health food stores. Start with a small dosage, and adjust it gradually until you find the amount suitable for you. Be sure to drink it with lots of water.

Bran is available as coarse miller's bran, or in convenient tablet form. Both forms are available in health food stores. As with psyllium, start with a small dosage: you may experience some gas and bloating when you first start out. Adjust the amount gradually over several weeks until you find the amount that's right for you.

Drink Lots Of Fluids

Water is essential to proper digestion and flushing out the system. I recommend a minimum of six to eight glasses of water and other fluids a day to prevent constipation.

Avoid Seeds And Hard Particles

Once you've developed diverticulosis, you should avoid seeds, nuts, and hard particles, such as popcorn, which can become lodged in the sacs of the colon and become infected, causing an attack of diverticulitis. Avoid poppy seeds and sesame seeds used in bakery toppings, or grain particles in cracked-wheat bread. Seeds found in vegetables and fruits, such as cucumbers or oranges or grapes, should also be avoided.

A Natural Treatment For Diverticular Disease

- Adopt a high fiber diet. That means lots of fruits and vegetables, whole grains, cereals, etc. Avoid eating processed food: substitute whole grain bread for white, a whole apple for apple juice.
- If you have trouble handling bran, take psyllium seed bulking agents. Follow the directions on the package and be sure to take with plenty of water.

- Drink plenty of fluids every day: from six to eight glass of water or other fluid.

- Avoid constipation and, if you do become constipated, don't use laxatives. If you experience some constipation, increase your psyllium and water intake and, if this doesn't work, add bran to your diet. You can take it in tablet form, available in health food stores. You take three tablets a day and increase by three tablets every few days until you achieve the desired result.

  You can also take bran in the form of coarse miller's bran. In that form, you take a tablespoon a day and increase it by a tablespoon every few days. You can also sprinkle it on foods and cereals or mix it into baked foods like muffins and meat-loaves. Increase bran intake gradually over the course of about a month. You can expect some gas and bloating when you first begin to take it. (See CONSTIPA-TION, page 143.)

- Avoid eating seeds, nuts and foods with hard particles that could become lodged in the diverticular sacs. These foods include strawberries, figs, tomatoes, zucchini, cucumber, baked goods that have cracked wheat, poppy, sesame or caraway seeds.

CHAPTER 15

Dry Skin

People who live in normally humid climates seldom have trouble with dry skin. But in dry climates, or in a centrally heated house or office, the dry air actually absorbs moisture from the skin, leaving it dry, flaky and uncomfortable. If the condition is not corrected, the skin becomes increasingly painful and tight. Eventually, it can crack open and become vulnerable to infection.

To correct the problem, you must humidify the air so that it's not depleting moisture from your skin. And you must protect the natural moisture of your skin by using a moisturizer or cream that will act as a protective barrier against further loss of moisture. In some cases, however, people develop red and irritated skin, not because of dryness, but because they're allergic to the moisturizer itself.

This happened to Sally, one of my regular patients. Sally, an assistant district attorney, was in her late thirties when she had her first child and took an extended leave of absence from her job. She came to see me six months later, in the spring. When she held out her hands I saw that they were red and inflamed, with small, painful-looking blisters around the fingertips.

"Housewife hands," she said cheerfully enough. "I've got my hands in water half the time," she added, "which is how they got so dry in the first place — and they're not getting better, even though I now use rubber gloves and tons of hand lotion."

Sally was right about water drying out her hands. Though it sounds like a contradiction, water is very drying to the skin, and soaps and detergents dry the skin out further. But Sally had been using rubber gloves without improvement, and the extreme irritation of her hands led me to suspect contact dermatitis.

I told Sally that I believed she was allergic to her hand lotion. Instead of sending her to an allergist, I recommended that she discontinue using the hand lotion for a week or two. Two weeks to the day, Sally called to tell me that the inflammation had cleared up, and the hand lotion was obviously to blame.

Unfortunately, many people don't realize that their red and irritated skin is due to the very moisturizers they are using to cure or prevent dryness. If you suspect you are allergic to a cleanser or cosmetic, discontinue their use for a week or so to see if the redness clears up — and then re-introduce them one at a time, until you isolate the offending product.

If, on the other hand, your dry skin is due to dry, heated air and too much exposure to water, the following guidelines will help you take corrective measures that will restore your skin to its normal, supple state.

Humidify The Air

If you consider that the ideal humidity for human skin is 30 to 40 percent, and the humidity level in the average heated house is 10 percent, you'll appreciate why your skin can become so dry and flaky. A cool-mist humidifier is the best way to combat this dryness and humidify the air in your home. Keep one on in your bedroom at night (one of my patients tells me that she turns it on as soon as she comes home from work, so that the room feels pleasant by the time she goes to bed) and another one in the living room or kitchen. Just remember to keep your humidifier clean: clean it carefully, following manufacturer's instructions at the beginning of the season and occasionally throughout the season.

Plants can also be effective in humidifying the air, and are particularly appropriate in an office, where a humidifier might be impractical. Decorative vases filled with water, on the windowsills or the radiators, are another way of adding moisture to the air.

Moisturize! Moisturize!

Adding a moisturizer to the surface of your skin will help hold in moisture and keep skin from drying out. The best time to apply moisturizer is when your skin is still slightly damp from your shower or bath. Also, keep some moisturizer on your kitchen and bathroom sinks, and apply some each time you wash and dry your hands.

You can experiment with various moisturizers until you find the one you like most. Just keep in mind that the best moisturizers are not necessarily the most expensive ones. For instance, Vaseline is one of the best and cheapest moisturizers around. Its disadvantage, of course, is that it can be too greasy. Use it at night, to protect your skin against loss of moisture: rub it on your hands, elbows, knees, etc. — any place that feels tight and dry. Another good nighttime moisturizer is Crisco, which doctors often recommend to people who've had procedures such as chemical peels.

For daytime use, you may prefer a lighter moisturizer. Some of my patients like Nivea or Lubriderm, and Sea Breeze Moisture Lotion has been highly rated by *Consumer Reports*.

The Best Moisturizers

Lotions containing lactic acid can be extremely helpful for severe dryness. Lac-Hydrin, which requires your doctor's prescription, actually changes the surface of your skin to allow it to retain additional moisture. Two other lotions which contain less lactic acid are available over-the-counter. They are called Lac-Hydrin Five and LactiCare, and they too are very effective for dry skin.

Another ointment popular with some people is Bag Balm, which is an udder ointment sold in farm supply stores. However, if you are allergic to wool, you may also be allergic to lanolin, which is an ingredient in Bag Balm. Other products that contain lanolin are Lanoline, A and D Ointment, and Keri.

Water Can Dry You Out!

Many people think that when their skin is dry a long, hot shower will moisturize it. Quite the contrary. Since water, particularly hot water, can be drying to the skin, limit the number of showers and baths you take, and use warm, rather than hot water, which has a stronger drying effect.

Another problem with the long, hot shower is that it usually means lots of soap. Soaps and many cleansers can be terribly drying to the skin, as well as irritating, so avoid using soaps and detergents that dry the skin further. Dove is known as a good, mild soap. Many people mistakenly think Ivory is mild, but it's really a strong, pure soap and thus drying. Ask your pharmacy or health food store for alternative cleansers you can use that will not be drying.

To further protect your hands, use rubber gloves whenever cleaning, washing dishes, or doing other kitchen preparations. You can get rubber gloves at the supermarket, or buy the disposable latex surgical gloves available at pharmacies or pet supply stores.

Improve Your Nutritional Status

Lack of adequate nutrients can result in overall dryness of the skin. I've noticed this problem particularly with women who have cut most of the fat from their diets. They complain about how dry their skin has become, forgetting that the body requires some fat in the diet in order to keep the skin moist and supple. If you have eliminated virtually all fat from your diet, try adding one or two tablespoonfuls of olive oil a day. You should notice improvement in just a few days.

Check Your Supplements

Zinc supplements in excess of 100 mg. a day can cause dry skin. Check your vitamin and mineral supplements to determine how much zinc you are taking, and reduce the amount to under 100 mg. a day.

A Natural Treatment For Dry Skin

- Be sure that your dry, reddened skin is not a case of contact dermatitis, especially if you've been using lots of different moisturizers. Use no moisturizers for a week or so (using other techniques listed below to help keep your skin moist) and if the redness clears up, you are allergic to something you've been using on your skin.

- Humidify the air with cool mist.

- Use Vaseline at night on dry areas.

- Use a moisturizer like Nivea or Lubiderm during the day.

- Try to use a moisturizer when your skin is damp to trap additional moisture.

- Protect hands from water using lined rubber gloves.

- Keep moisturizer on the sink to use each time you dry your hands.

- Severe dryness problems can be solved with prescription Lac Hydrin cream that actually changes the surface of the skin to help it retain moisture.

- Over-the-counter preparations like Lac-Hydrin Five and LactiCare can help dry skin.

- Bag Balm can be helpful for dry skin but be sure you don't have an allergy to lanolin, one of its principal ingredients.
- Bathe or shower only as needed.
- Use warm, not hot water.
- If dryness is severe, use a non-drying soap alternative like Cetaphil for cleansing.
- If you are on an extremely low fat diet, add one or two tablespoons of olive oil to your daily diet.
- If you are taking doses of zinc in excess of 100 mg. daily, reduce that amount.

CHAPTER 16

Fibrocystic Breast Disease

Fibrocystic breast disease is misnamed in that it's not really a disease, but a condition — also known as cystic mastitis — suffered by 60 percent of all women. Women with cystic mastitis experience swollen, cystic, or lumpy breasts, usually before a menstrual period. The condition is not medically dangerous, but it can be uncomfortable and painful.

Cindy, a bank executive in her mid-thirties, was typical of patients with cystic mastitis in that her breasts became so tender and swollen that she had trouble sleeping at night.

"They get so painful that even the touch of a sheet is irritating," she told me. "And it's not much better in the daytime, which makes it hard to concentrate on my work. And I have to drink a quart of coffee just to get me going. And there's another problem. . ." Cindy's expression became fearful. "Every time I feel a lump, I'm afraid of cancer. It's making me very anxious. Is there any medication you can give me?"

I told Cindy there were no effective medications for fibrocystic breast disease — but that natural therapy can alleviate the condition dramatically. I also explained to her how important it was to have regular mammograms: while the cysts that cause the discomfort of fibrocystic breast disease are entirely benign, they can sometimes mask lumps which could signal a problem. This is nothing to be overly concerned about but it is important that a woman who suffers from fibrocystic breast disease consult regularly with her gynecologist for expert examinations and regular mammograms.

Causes Of Cystic Mastitis

The onset of cystic mastitis appears to be regulated by estrogen, which is why the inflammatory process becomes most evident before a menstrual period. Both natural estrogen and the estrogen in birth control pills can have an effect on breasts with a tendency to cystic mastitis. (See **PMS**, page 311, for more information on this.) But diet also plays a significant role, and changes in the diet can provide almost total remission of all symptoms.

The first thing she should do, I told Cindy, is give up caffeine. That meant all coffee and caffeinated colas, as well tea and chocolate which contain a substance related to caffeine. She should also check her medications — such as those for asthma or allergies, for caffeine — and select alternative ones if caffeine was included.

While some studies appeared to show that caffeine reduction was not effective in controlling cystic fibrosis, they did not assess the effect of totally eliminating caffeine from the diet. My patients who have given up all caffeine and related substances have noticed a definite improvement in their condition.

I also told Cindy she should avoid meat and animal fats, which can prevent the excretion of inflammatory estrogens that contribute to the problem. Instead, she should eat a diet rich in fruits and vegetables, which would help to purge her system of detoxified estrogens and regulate her bowel function.

Constipation and irregular bowel movements can create a problem for women who tend toward cystic breasts. There is evidence that women who have fewer than three bowel movements a week are four and half times more likely to have cystic mastitis than women who move their bowels every day.

Seafood, rich in iodine, is also a desirable nutrient for women with cystic mastitis. Some animal studies have shown a link between iodine deficiency and cystic mastitis, and some doctors have had good results prescribing kelp supplements for their patients. Of course, your doctor would want to test you for thyroid activity before prescribing a supplement, but if your iodine is low because you are eating less iodized salt, seafood is a healthy way to supplement the deficiency.

There are a number of supplements, including vitamin E, vitamin A, and primrose oil, which have yielded dramatic results in controlling cystic fibrosis, and I recommended them to Cindy.

The Importance Of Mammograms

I also reminded her that she should get regular mammograms. As I mentioned earlier, Cindy had explained how each month, when she did a breast self-examination, she worried that one of the many lumps she felt in her breast might be cancerous.

Many patients with cystic mastitis have this concern, a legitimate one, because — though the condition is not in any way a precursor to cancer — it's difficult to distinguish the lumps of cystic mastitis from a new, and potentially malignant, lump. I believe that a mammogram is essential for all patients with cystic fibrosis, particularly if there is a history of cancer.

Get Some Support . . .

If you have fibrocystic breasts that become painful, particularly before your period, it can be very helpful to wear a good support bra. A jogging or sports bra which is comfortable but supportive can ease your discomfort, and many women find that wearing one even when sleeping gives great relief.

Cindy followed my natural therapy, and experienced almost total relief from her symptoms within a couple of months. If you have severe fibrocystic breast disease and do not experience sufficient relief from the natural therapy guidelines below, ask your doctor about iodine supplements, which have yielded excellent results.

Caffeine Is A Culprit

Caffeine can have a major effect on fibrocystic breasts and many women who eliminate caffeine from their diets find almost complete relief from the condition. Give up coffee and caffeinated colas. Check your medications for caffeine. Give up tea, which contains theophylline, related to caffeine, and chocolate, which contains theobromine.

You can substitute herbal teas, which do not contain caffeine. If you are used to drinking lots of cola drinks, remember to substitute water and/or water with a spritz of fruit juice in your daily routine. Some women give up colas and don't compensate for the fluid loss which causes them to become constipated.

Improve Your Nutritional Status

Since fibrocystic breast disease is an inflammatory condition, your body's reaction to your diet will affect the degree of the inflammatory process. Eat a diet high in fresh vegetables and fiber to encourage regular bowel movements and promote the excretion of detoxified estrogens. Avoid animal fats. Eat fish and other seafood rich in iodine. Follow the guidelines in a HEALTHY WOMAN'S DAILY ROUTINE, page 19.

Nutritional Supplements For Fibrocystic Breast Disease

Vitamin E is extremely effective in controlling cystic mastitis. In one study, 85 percent of the patients taking vitamin E had remission of the symptoms, and the other 15 percent showed improvement. Buy the natural vitamin E, which was used in the study. The synthetic vitamin E was found ineffective.

High doses of vitamin A are also effective in reducing the symptoms of cystic mastitis, but since it may produce headaches in some people, I recommend beta-carotene, with a similar effect, to my patients.

Primrose oil has been used effectively in Europe to treat the inflammation of cystic mastitis, and many of my patients have found it helpful in easing their symptoms.

Iodine supplements have been effective for people whose symptoms are resistant to natural therapy, but they require medical supervision because of potential side effects. Talk to your doctor about iodine supplements: he will want to test you for thyroid activity before making a decision.

A Natural Treatment For
Fibrocystic Breast Disease

- Eliminate coffee, tea, chocolate and caffeinated sodas from your diet. Check labels on over-the-counter medications because many diet preparations, analgesics, pain relievers, diuretics, cold and allergy remedies contain caffeine. Also, prescription drugs can contain caffeine. Check any you may take regularly.

- Avoid animal fats.

- Eat lots of fresh fruits, vegetables, nuts and berries.

- Eat fish and other seafood rich in iodine.

In addition to your daily basic antioxidant vitamin/mineral supplement, take:

- Vitamin E: 600 I.U. a day.

- Beta-carotene: 50,000 I.U.'s a day.

- Kelp: 6 tablets a day.

- Primrose oil: one or two capsules three times a day.

Also:

- Get regular mammograms.

- Ask your doctor if iodine supplements could be appropriate for you.

CHAPTER 17

Gallbladder Disease

Isabel, an Englishwoman visiting relatives in this country, was a textbook example of the suddenness of a gallbladder attack. When her relative, an old patient of mine, brought her to my office, Isabel was clearly in pain, holding herself hunched over, her face shiny with sweat. She was a pleasant looking woman in her late twenties, but overweight, I estimated, by as much as thirty or forty pounds. She gave me a brave smile.

"Actually, it seems to be getting better," she said. "It was worse during the night — isn't it always? — and I thought I was dying of appendicitis. Or a bleeding ulcer, maybe."

The pain of a gallbladder attack can be extreme and many patients only become aware they are suffering from gallbladder disease after they are stricken with this pain which they, understandably, often mistake for something like appendicitis or an ulcer. Indeed, in the past the approach to gallbladder disease was to wait until the pain became almost intolerable and then to remove the gallbladder. Today we have other, better, alternatives.

The gallbladder, which is located under the liver and just behind the bottom right rib, is used to store bile, a substance produced by the liver to help in the digestion of fat. Gallbladder disease is most frequently associated with a diet high in cholesterol and refined carbohydrates. When you eat fatty foods, the bile becomes saturated with cholesterol. Eventually, this excess cholesterol may cause inflammation of the gallbladder, or may separate from the bile and begin to calcify, forming stones. In the United States, 80 percent of gallbladder stones are formed from excessive cholesterol, while the remaining twenty percent are formed from various minerals.

People with gallstones may remain symptom-free, often for years. Others may suffer from intermittent symptoms of indigestion such as gas, bloating, and nausea, particularly after they eat a meal rich in animal-saturated fats. The discomfort is similar whether they have gallstones, or an inflamed gallbladder as yet free of stones. But the pain can become severe when a stone starts to travel from the gallbladder into one of the bile ducts leading to the liver.

When I examined Isabel, she pointed to the upper right corner of her abdomen to show me the location of her pain. I told Isabel that she was experiencing a gallbladder attack, and a sonogram confirmed the presence of gallstones.

Most gallbladder attacks are transient: they peak after several hours, and then gradually fade away when the stone had passed. Subsequent attacks may be more severe, and the recovery period takes longer. Eventually, gallbladder disease may progress to an acute gallbladder attack due to an obstructive stone that doesn't clear, or to a severe inflammation of the gallbladder wall.

Techniques For Removing Gallstones

When Isabel asked me what her options were, I told her that many doctors recommend surgery to prevent further gallbladder attacks. The advent of laparoscopic surgery, which requires very small incisions, has reduced the risk and recovery time associated at one time with surgical removal of the gallbladder. As a consequence, the number of gallbladder surgical procedures has almost doubled. But the surgery is still not risk-free, and many patients who have had surgery are dismayed to find their symptoms return when new stones form within the bile ducts, or the bile ducts become inflamed!

Other techniques for eliminating gallstones include a drug that dissolves them, and shock-wave lithotripsy that pulverizes them. These techniques have advantages and disadvantages that should be discussed with your individual doctors, but, as I told Isabel, in both cases the stones and the inflammation may return.

Natural Alternatives For Gallbladder Disease

Natural therapy was the treatment I recommended for Isabel. It wouldn't eliminate her gallbladder stones, but it would keep her free from further gallbladder disease symptoms, and — just as important — by following dietary guidelines she would improve her overall health by reducing her high cholesterol count and obesity.

I gave Isabel my guidelines for controlling gallbladder disease, and did not see her again. But I did get a postcard from England four months later. She had written: "Did what you recommended. Never felt better. Isabel."

Gallbladder disease is more frequent in women than in men, and appears to target special ethnic groups, including the English — such as Isabel — as well as Asians, Indians, and Latin Americans.

If you have a history of gallbladder disease in your family, or have experienced gas, bloating, or indigestion following a high cholesterol meal, you should follow the natural therapy guidelines to keep from developing chronic or acute attacks of gallbladder disease.

Diet And Gallbladder Disease

The first, and most effective thing you can do to avoid gallstones, or prevent a gallbladder attack, is to eliminate foods that are high in fat and cholesterol. A high fat meal causes your gallbladder to release extra bile: the higher the fat content, the more bile is required. In the process, a stone may be released or the walls of the gallbladder may become inflamed.

Since research indicates that low fiber diets are also implicated in gallbladder disease, increase the fiber in your diet, particularly water soluble fiber found in vegetables and fruits, pectin, and oat bran.

There are also indications that women who skip breakfast, or have only coffee for breakfast, are also increasing their potential to develop gallstones.

In addition, drink adequate liquids — a minimum of six to eight glasses of water a day — so that you have the necessary fluids to maintain the water content of the bile and prevent the formation of stones.

For additional information on a proper diet, refer to A HEALTHY WOMAN'S DAILY ROUTINE, page 19.

There was a very recent report in <u>The Lancet</u>, a respected British medical journal, that made a connection between fair-skinned people who suntan and gallstones. People in general who enjoy sunbathing have twice the risk of gallstones; fair-skinned people who sunbathe run twenty times the risk of non-sunbathers for developing gallstones. This research is in its preliminary stages but it's information that could be significant for people who are troubled by gallstones.

Check For Food Allergies

As far back as 1948, Dr. J. C. Breneman, who had done extensive work with food allergies, reported that allergenic foods stimulated the swelling of the bile ducts, thus reducing the flow of bile and causing the pain and other symptoms of a gallbladder attack. He developed a successful regime to eliminate gallbladder attacks by eliminating allergens from the diet.

In one study, 100 percent of gallbladder patients were totally free of symptoms when they followed a basic allergy elimination diet. The foods that most often produced allergic reactions were eggs (93 percent of the patients reacted to eggs), pork, onions, fowl, milk, coffee, citrus, corn, beans, and nuts. Allergies explain why some patients who have had gallbladder surgery continue to suffer from recurring attacks.

Try an allergy elimination diet to see if it will also eliminate your gallbladder symptoms, and gradually reintroduce the various food categories, watching each one for possible reactions.

Lose Weight . . . Sensibly

Overweight is a strong predictor of gallbladder problems, and if you are overweight you add to your odds of developing gallbladder disease with every pound. For instance, if you are 20 percent overweight, your risk of developing gallstones is doubled. The high fiber, low fat diets recommended for gallbladder patients will also help you lose weight. However, avoid the "protein" crash diets, which recent research has shown can actually promote the development of gallstones.

Try Aspirin

There is indication that aspirin may inhibit the production of stones. In one study, for instance, 32 percent of the patients who did not use aspirin regularly had a recurrence of gallstones, while none of the patients who used NSAID's had a recurrence. I recommend a daily baby aspirin to my gallbladder patients.

Nutritional Supplements For Gallbladder Disease

Calcium, a mineral that is essential to the health of women's bones, can also be helpful in preventing gallbladder disease. A recent study of 860 men provided new evidence that calcium intake reduces the formation of gallstones, possibly by changing the formation of the bile.

Lecithin is another nutritional supplement that can help gallstone patients by preventing excess cholesterol from separating from the bile and forming gallstones.

A Natural Treatment For Gallbladder Disease

- Eliminate any possible food allergies. If you need help in determining whether or not you have such allergies, consult with a doctor trained in nutritional therapy.
- Avoid aggravating foods which include all fatty foods and fried foods. See A HEALTHY WOMAN'S DAILY ROUTINE,

page 19, for more information on eliminating fat from the diet.

- Increase your fiber intake, particularly eating more of the following foods: fruits, vegetables, whole grain breads and cereals and oat bran.

- If you are overweight, lose weight on a sensible diet. Do *not* go on an extremely low-calorie diet as this can exacerbate gallstones.

- Be sure to drink 6 to 8 glasses of water daily.

- Eat a healthy breakfast daily.

- Avoid caffeine.

In addition to your daily basic antioxidant vitamin/mineral supplement, take:

- Lecithin: 500 mg. three times a day.

> Surgery is the traditional route for gallstones that are persistent and troublesome. But there are some new techniques that are being used in lieu of conventional surgery. There is a drug that dissolves stones; there is a new surgical technique using laparoscopic (microsurgical) techniques that require small incisions; there is shock wave lithotripsy which "crushes" the stones. These techniques have their advantages and disadvantages and should be discussed with your doctor.

CHAPTER 18

Heavy Periods

Rhoda, a thin energetic woman in her mid-forties, looked rushed and harried when she came into my office. She had come to see me as a last-ditch measure before getting a hysterectomy, she said. She didn't want the surgery, but as a clinical psychologist with a busy practice she couldn't afford the inconvenience of the heavy periods that were forcing her to stay home each month. Did I have any suggestions?

Heavy periods, or menorrhagia, affect many women of menstruating age and, though they are seldom a cause of concern, they can prove to be a major inconvenience. Some women suffering from heavy periods put off seeing a gynecologist because they are afraid they have cancer, but heavy periods in premenopausal women are seldom indicative of cancer.

If you are experiencing excessively heavy bleeding during your period, or if the period lasts longer than five days, you should visit your gynecologist to rule out organic causes, such as cysts or fibroids. An intrauterine device (IUD) can also cause excessive menstrual bleeding.

Rhoda told me she had been given a clean bill of health by the gynecologist. She had been told, however, that the only two ways to control her heavy bleeding were to resume the contraceptive pills she had recently discontinued taking, or have a hysterectomy. Since she didn't want to use hormone therapy — she felt that after fifteen years on the pill her body needed a rest — her one remaining option was the hysterectomy, a major surgical procedure from which it would take her several weeks to recover.

Fortunately, I was able to tell Rhoda about some natural supplements that proved helpful for her heavy periods. If you bleed excessively during your periods, or have periods that last longer than five days, try the following natural treatments before considering more drastic therapies such as hormone supplements or a hysterectomy.

First, Get A Gynecological Exam

See your gynecologist to make sure there is no organic cause for your heavy periods.

Try Nutritional Supplements

Women who have heavy periods may be deficient in vitamin A. It has been established that women with heavy periods have lower doses of vitamin A than women with normal periods. The levels of vitamin A go up while you are on the pill, and go back down once the pill is discontinued. I've had several patients who, like Rhoda, started having heavy periods after they stopped taking the pill. Take a vitamin A supplement with your meals.

Bioflavonoids, which are found in the inner peel and the white pulp of citrus fruit, are helpful in maintaining strong blood vessels. Take a bioflavonoid supplement twice daily.

Vitamin C is also important in maintaining strong tissue and blood vessels. Take a vitamin C supplement twice daily.

Ask you doctor to do a blood test to determine if you are anemic. Heavy periods can cause iron deficiency anemia, and iron deficiency, in turn, can cause heavy periods. If your blood test shows that you are anemic, take a daily dose of elemental iron with your meals.

Since low levels of zinc have also been implicated with heavy periods, take a zinc supplement with meals.

Suspend The Use Of Vitamin E And Aspirin

Both vitamin E and aspirin have an impact on blood clotting. In fact, people who take vitamin E and aspirin sometimes report that they bleed and bruise easily. Stop taking vitamin E and aspirin for a month or two to determine if your bleeding decreases.

A Natural Treatment For Heavy Periods

- Check with your doctor to see that there is no organic cause for your heavy periods such as a tumor (including fibroid tumor), cysts, I.U.D.s, etc.

In addition to your daily basic antioxidant vitamin/mineral supplement, take:

- Vitamin A: Take 25,000 I.U. daily for three months, then 10,000 I.U.
- Bioflavonoids and Vitamin C: Take 1000 mg. of bioflavonoids plus an equal amount of vitamin C twice a day.
- Iron: If a blood test has revealed that you are anemic, take 100 mg. daily with meals. (Iron can cause constipation and/or dark bowel movements.)
- Zinc: 50 mg. a day with meals.

Also:

- Discontinue both Vitamin E and aspirin for a month or two to see if your periods become less heavy.

CHAPTER 19

Hemorrhoids

Unfortunately, hemorrhoids are one of those health problems that can be as embarrassing to some women as they are uncomfortable. If you do suffer from hemorrhoids, know that roughly eighty percent of your fellow Americans have suffered along with you; they are one of our most common health problems.

Hemorrhoids are veins located in the anus which have become stretched and weakened, usually as a result of straining to eliminate dry and hard stools. They are virtually unknown in undeveloped countries, and are largely a result of our Western diet, which promotes constipation because it is so limited in fiber. Once hemorrhoids develop, they can be aggravated by other activities which cause pressure or straining, such as sitting, heavy lifting, or pregnancy and childbirth.

Valerie, as many other patients with hemorrhoids, had been bothered by pain and itching in her rectal area, but she didn't come to see me until she noticed fresh, red blood in her stool. Frightened, she assumed that she had developed some type of cancer. I examined her to confirm that hemorrhoids were the problem, and explained to Valerie that the bleeding was caused when the veins, already weakened from straining, had been abraded by the pressure of a hard, dry stool during elimination.

Valerie was also typical of most patients with hemorrhoids in that she was eating a diet high in animal fats and refined carbohydrates, and low in fresh fruits, vegetables and legumes that are high in fiber. A financial analyst who spent long days in front of a computer screen, Valerie was in the habit of sending out for a sandwich at lunch, and picking up a pizza or Chinese take-out for dinner. She frequently took laxatives for her constipation, which only made things worse, because, in the long run, laxatives actually promote constipation. She had also started using some over-the-counter remedies for hemorrhoids which were providing some limited topical relief, but no long-term solution.

I told Valerie she could eliminate her hemorrhoids by taking natural supplements and making some basic changes to her diet, an approach that would promote her overall good health. I gave her my dietetic guidelines and explained that, by avoiding a diet that promoted constipation, she would also avoid more serious health problems, such diverticular disease. I also suggested she take "sitz" baths to shrink the veins and reduce the inflammation, and use topical ointments for immediate relief.

I've had great success in helping patients over-come their problems with hemorrhoids, and Valerie was no exception. Within a few weeks her hemor-rhoids had cleared up, and to date they have not re-turned.

If you are suffering from hemmorrhoids, the fol-lowing guidelines will give you quick relief, and will help you to avoid the condition in the future.

To Relieve Your Symptoms. . .

Use a topical ointment to obtain quick — though temporary — relief. While there are numer-ous over-the-counter products for hemmorrhoids, you can do as well — and spend less — by buying zinc oxide, petroleum jelly, or witch hazel. Dab one of these products over the affected area regularly until your discomfort subsides.

> Note: Over-the-counter remedies that claim to shrink tissue must carry a warning because people with certain health problems, including heart disease and diabetes, should not use them. Avoid these products if you have any of the conditions listed in the warning.

A sitz bath, which involves sitting in three or four inches of warm water with your knees raised, can also provide you with quick relief by drawing blood to the area, and shrinking the painful veins.

If your job requires long periods of sitting in a chair or a car, buy an inflatable donut — a sort of balloon you sit on that takes pressure off the rectal area — at the pharmacy to provide relief.

Don't irritate already painful veins by using harsh toilet tissue. Instead, buy premoistened towelettes — those without added ingredients that can act as irritants — and use them to soothe and avoid additional irritation.

Improve Your Nutritional Status

To cure your hemorrhoids, rather than merely relieve the symptoms, you must change your diet. A soft and bulky stool is easier to eliminate without straining, and can be achieved through a high fiber diet. This means a diet high in fruits, whole grains, legumes and vegetables.

Don't make a changeover overnight, however, because this could cause you diarrhea. Do it gradually, over a week or two, replacing the refined carbohydrates in your diet with fruits and vegetables. I don't recommend the use of bran supplements for additional roughage, because bran can become irritating to delicate tissue.

If your dietary changes don't produce a sufficiently soft and bulky stool, you can add a bulking agent, such as psyllium, which attracts and holds water to create a softer, larger stool.

Whether or not you take psyllium, be sure to increase your water consumption. You should take eight glasses of water a day. Since many people forget to keep track of how much they're drinking, I recommend a simple means of keeping score. Put eight pennies in your pocket when you get dressed in the morning, and, each time you drink a glass of water, switch a penny over to your other pocket.

Since alcohol, coffee and nuts can be irritating to hemorrhoids, eliminate them from your diet if you notice additional irritation after eating them.

For additional information about a balanced diet, refer to A HEALTHY WOMAN'S DAILY ROUTINE, page 19.

Try Nutritional Supplements

Rutin, part of the C complex, is a bioflavonoid that strengthens the capillary system. It has been of great help to some of my patients who suffer from hemorrhoids. Try adding a rutin supplement to your diet.

A Natural Treatment For Hemorrhoids

- For immediate relief, apply a topical over-the-counter ointment or simply use zinc oxide, petroleum jelly or witch hazel. Dab on the affected area regularly until symptoms are relieved.
- Take two or three sitz baths daily: sit in a warm bath with your knees raised for five to fifteen minutes.

- If you must sit for long periods of time, or if you simply need immediate relief from painful hemorrhoids, buy a "doughnut" at your pharmacy and use it to sit on to relieve the pressure of the hemmhorhoids.

- Shift the emphasis of your diet to high fiber, complex carbohdyrate foods. Gradually increase the amounts of fruits, vegetables, whole grain breads, beans and other high fiber foods. Gradually eliminate highly refined foods.

- Use a stool softener or psyllium powder — 1 teaspoon in water once or twice daily when you first notice symptoms, or if hard stool is not relieved by diet.

- Take rutin: 100 milligrams, three times a day.

- Improve your bowel habits. Don't strain; move your bowels only when you feel the urge. Limit the time you spend on the toilet — don't use the bathroom as a library!

- Don't use harsh toilet paper. Use premoistened towelettes and wipe gently.

- Avoid lifting heavy objects as this puts a stress on your circulatory system.

- If you are pregnant, it can help to lie down on your left side and rest for about a half-hour two or three times a day. It also helps to lie on your left side at night, if you're comfortable in that position, to relieve the pressure of the fetus on the vein serving the lower half of the body.

If, after a period of time, you find that an improved diet, use of a stool softener, better bowel habits and topical applications to relieve symptoms don't solve your problem, it is possible that you will need surgery. Surgical techniques for hemorrhoids are relatively simple today; consult with your doctor.

CHAPTER 20

Herpes

While genital herpes is the most common venereal disease in the United States, it is neither dangerous nor life-threatening except to newborn infants. But Annette, a patient suffering from herpes, was clearly terrified. She was a tall, fair-skinned, freckled girl in her late teens, and as she stood in the middle of my office chewing on her knuckles I thought she looked even younger than her age.

"My infection has flared up again, and I don't know how I'm going to tell my boyfriend," she said, and started to cry.

Annette's story was similar to that of many other patients with herpes. Several years ago, while still in high school, she had sex with a boy she met at a party: she had too much to drink, and felt woozy, and it just happened, she said.

A few days later she was dismayed to find a rash on her buttocks and genital area. The doctor she consulted told her it was genital herpes, and warned her there might be recurrent flare-ups in the future. But the sores cleared up within three weeks, and there had been no recurrence for two years. Until now. What made it so bad is that she had met this terrific boy in college, and things were getting sort of serious between them. Was there anything I could do to help her? she said.

Unfortunately, there is no cure for herpes, I told Annette, though we can mitigate its effects and reduce the odds of recurrence.

Herpes is caused by the herpes simplex virus, one of the large family of herpesvirus, which cause all sorts of ailments, from shingles to chickenpox. There are two variations of herpes simplex. Type 1 is associated with sores around the mouth, and type 2 affects the genitalia — blisters and sores on the penis and scrotum on men, and the vulva on women. The buttocks and thighs may also be affected.

The two types of herpes virus can be interchangeable, so that oral sex with a partner who has an active cold sore may well cause an infection of the genitalia. After the initial infection, the herpes virus lies dormant in the nerves, and is not infectious during its dormant stage. But periodically, the infection is likely to flare up again, and is infectious to a sexual partner until it abates again. It has been estimated that the odds of infection as a result of sexual contact during an active outbreak of herpes are as high as 75 percent.

Obviously, it is the responsibility of anyone with herpes to inform a potential sexual partner and to abstain from sex during an outbreak. Unfortunately, this is not always done, and the problem is complicated by the fact that both women and men may have a painless, though still infectious outbreak with no visible sores. There are approximately twenty million Americans with herpes, and an additional half a million are infected every year.

Annette, who had been infected by a callously thoughtless sexual partner, told me she had not had a sexual encounter since that time. She had, however, thought she was cured of the herpes infection, and had planned on having intercourse with her boyfriend when they both felt the time was right. Now she would have to tell him, and he would probably want to break off the relationship, she said. She was no longer crying, but her woebegone expression spoke volumes.

It's always very difficult to find out you have a disease for which there is, as yet, no cure. Fortunately, herpes simplex is not, as a rule, dangerous to the people who have it, except to newborns infected with the disease, for whom the infection may be fatal. Since a baby may pick up the infection as it travels through the birth canal of a mother with an active outbreak, most obstetricians will recommend a "C" section to women with an active infection at the time of delivery.

I told Annette that, while we couldn't eradicate the virus from her system, there were several things she could do to boost her immune system and prevent outbreaks in the future. Many of my patients have found that by modifying their diet, taking certain key supplements, and avoiding stress, they could effectively prevent future outbreaks. I also gave Annette some basic guidelines for gaining immediate relief from her symptoms, and asked her to call me in a couple of weeks to let me know how she was doing.

When she did call a few days later, I could tell she was smiling just by hearing her voice. "It's all right," she told me. "No, I don't mean the rash, though that's almost cleared up. I was talking about my boyfriend — I told him, and he still is. My boyfriend, that is."

Two years after that first visit, Annette came to see me about another matter and I questioned her about her herpes. She told me that she had had only one recurrence in the two years since she began treatment and it was just before her marriage. She had gone on to marry that boyfriend but it could have been the stress of preparing for the wedding that precipitated her bout with herpes. At any rate, she did find that following my recommendations, particularly those concerning stress control, were truly effective in keeping herpes outbreaks at bay.

Shown below are basic guidelines for what to do for a herpes infection, and a program designed to avoid future outbreaks.

Treating The Symptoms Of A Herpes Infection

If you're exposed to herpes and have indeed developed the infection, you will notice the symptoms within four or five days. These may range from pain, itching and sores at the site of contact, to flulike symptoms such as fever, headache, muscle aches, and fatigue. I recommend that you call your doctor immediately to request the antiviral drug acyclovir (Zovirax) which shortens the symptoms of the first attack, usually the worst. Subsequent flare-ups are much milder and seldom require acyclovir.

Avoid Spreading the Infection. . .

To keep the infection from spreading to other parts of your body, do not touch the affected area and then touch your eyes, face or mouth. Wash your hands with anti-bacterial soap after touching the active lesions.

It's important to keep the herpes blisters clean and dry. Wash them with soap and water. Some of my patients told me that drying their genitals with a hair dryer on low heat feels soothing. Do not use ointments or creams which will delay the drying action. Wear cotton underwear, and avoid tight, binding clothes to give your skin a chance to "breathe." An ice pack applied for ten minutes on, and five minutes off, may provide some relief.

A Caution. . .

Never use a cortisone cream on an active herpes outbreak as it can actually slow your immune response to the herpes attack and encourage the virus to grow. In addition, don't use any heavy creams like petroleum jelly as they can slow the healing process by keeping air from the herpes lesions.

Stress And Herpes: The Critical Link

Stress is a major stimulant of herpes outbreaks. You cannot eliminate the stress in your life but I believe that it's critical for you to take steps to control that stress. For more information on this, see STRESS CONTROL, page 321. I tell all my herpes patients they must adopt the relaxation response exercise described in that chapter and they must do it at least twice a day. Many have reported fewer outbreaks when following this regime.

Nutritional Therapy For Herpes

Certain nutrients can help prevent herpes outbreaks. Beta-carotene strengthens the immune system and can help inhibit viruses. Both vitamin C and zinc are helpful in inhibiting herpes attacks. And finally, vitamin E has been shown to be helpful in relieving the pain of the herpes outbreak and also in shortening the duration of the attack.

A Helpful Supplement

In my experience, the most effective aid in the relief of herpes is the amino acid L-lysine. There is a hypothesis that lysine inhibits herpes activity (while another amino acid, arginine, promotes it). And studies have demonstrated that lysine treatment can be very beneficial to herpes sufferers.

A maintenance dosage can be taken as a preventive and then increased if you experience an outbreak of the infection. If you take lysine supplements, be sure to watch your cholesterol levels as there's some evidence that lysine may stimulate the liver to increase production of cholesterol.

In addition to taking lysine as a supplement, it can be applied topically in the form of lysine cream, available in health food stores. I usually advise applying it topically twice a day but check with the directions on the label of the package.

Following the hypothesis that herpes outbreaks are stimulated by the imbalance of the amino acids arginine and lysine, it can also be beneficial to avoid arginine-containing foods while taking the lysine supplements. The foods to avoid include chocolate, peanuts and other nuts, seeds and cereal grains.

Yogurt To The Rescue

Lactobacillus acidophilus, the living culture used to make yogurt and acidophilus, can be helpful in fighting herpes. It can help relieve the symptoms of an outbreak as well as prevent future outbreaks. You can find lactobacillus acidophilus in capsule form in health food stores. Be sure to buy capsules that contain living cultures. They are usually kept refrigerated.

A Natural Treatment For Genital Herpes

For Immediate Relief. . .

- At the first signs of an initial outbreak — pain, burning and itching at the site of contact 4 to 5 days after encounter with infected partner — call your doctor to confirm diagnosis and get a prescription for acyclovir (Zovirax) which will lessen the severity of the initial outbreak.

In addition to your daily basic antioxidant vitamin/mineral supplement, take:

- L-lysine: 3000 milligrams daily; 1000 milligrams with each meal at the first sign of a cold sore outbreak. After the symptoms lessen, reduce your intake to 500 milligrams a day. If you break out on this maintenance dosage, increase your maintenance dose to 1000 milligrams a day to prevent recurrence.
- Lactobacillus acidophilus: 3 capsules a day, one with each meal.
- Zinc: 22.5–50 milligrams a day.
- Vitamin C with bioflavonoids: 1000–2000 milligrams a day.
- Vitamin E: 400 I.U.

Also

- Lysine cream: apply topically to lesions twice a day or as recommended on label.
- Keep affected area clean and dry.
- Do not use over-the-counter ointments or creams on the lesions, unless prescribed by a doctor.
- To keep the area dry, wear cotton underwear and non-binding clothes.
- Warm baths — two or three daily during an outbreak — can give relief.
- Relief from pain can be achieved with the use of an ice pack or ice covered with a clean cloth. Apply to lesions for ten minutes and then remove for five minutes. Repeat three or four times.
- Remember not to touch the lesions and then touch your fact, mouth, eyes, as this can spread the infection.

To Control Future Outbreaks. . .

- Adopt a method of stress control. See STRESS CONTROL, page 321.

Avoid arginine-rich foods, including:

- Chocolate
- Peanuts and other nuts
- Seeds
- Cereal grains, such as oatmeal
- Gelatin
- Carob
- Raisins

For More Help. . .

Three sources for additional help and information are:

The Herpes Hotline: (415) 328-7710, Monday through Friday, 12 to 4:30 P.M. (Pacific time).

STD Hotline: 1-800-227-8922, Monday through Friday, 5 A.M. to 8 P.M. (Pacific time).

The National Herpes Hotline: (919) 361-8488 (a recording).

CHAPTER 21

Hypertension

Marissa was stunned when she learned that she had high blood pressure, or hypertension. An energetic, fashionably dressed woman in her mid-fifties, Marissa is an account executive with one of the largest advertising firms in the country, a demanding job that she clearly enjoys. "I can still hardly believe it," Marissa told me of her doctor's diagnosis. "I had no idea there was anything wrong. In fact, I've never felt better."

Most people experience no symptoms from high blood pressure until it has caused major damage to their organs and circulatory system, which is why it's been called "the silent killer." There are 60 million people with hypertension in this country, which makes the condition a major medical challenge. People with hypertension have three times the risk of heart attack and seven times the risk of stroke as do people with normal blood pressure.

Fortunately, high blood pressure is easily diagnosed during a medical checkup, and there are several drugs available to reduce blood pressure to near normal levels. But Marissa had heard that these drugs had side effects which included fatigue and depression, and before starting treatment she was eager to explore other alternatives.

I told Marissa that natural measures can be of enormous help in controlling hypertension. Most of my patients have been able to reduce their medication following natural therapy, and many were able to eliminate it altogether. I questioned Marissa closely about her medical history, and conducted an examination to determine the extent of her hypertension.

There are two types of hypertension. Primary, or essential hypertension accounts for 85 to 90 percent of all cases, and its cause is not known, although heredity may predispose some individuals to it. Secondary hypertension, on the other hand, is due to a specific cause, such as a tumor or kidney disease, and returns to normal once the disease is treated. According to her doctor's diagnosis, Marissa was suffering from primary hypertension.

There are many degrees of hypertension, of course, ranging from borderline to severe. Since blood pressure varies considerably during the day — lower when you are at rest, and higher after activity or excitement — most doctors will do repeated readings before arriving at a diagnosis of hypertension.

Some people, in fact, experience "white coat syndrome," which means that the experience of being in a doctor's office is enough to elevate their blood pressure! Certain drugs can also distort a reading by temporarily elevating blood pressure. Phenylpropanolamine (PPA) for example, which is the active ingredient in various over-the-counter drugs including decongestants, cold remedies, and appetite suppressants, can elevate your pressure, and so can caffeine. A decongestant and two cups of coffee an hour before your checkup can produce an alarmingly elevated reading.

What Do Those Numbers Mean?

Blood pressure is the force exerted by the blood against the arterial blood vessels, and a blood pressure reading has two numbers. The first number, generally the higher one, measures the systolic pressure, which is the pressure when the heart contracts to pump the blood. The second number, the diastolic pressure, represents the pressure when the heart is resting in between contractions.

Marissa had a reading in the mild high blood pressure category, and had an excellent chance of bringing her pressure under control with natural therapy. She was very relieved to hear it, because she had been reading about hypertension, and was confused about when — and by how much — hypertension should be reduced by means of medication. I told her she wasn't the only one to be confused. As it turns out, there's been a great deal of controversy within the medical profession on the topic.

Here is how the National Institutes of Health currently classify the appropriate response to blood pressure readings:

SYSTOLIC PRESSURE
(If diastolic pressure below 90)

Less than 140: normal. Recheck within two years.

140-159: borderline isolated systolic hypertension. Confirm within two months.

160 or higher: isolated systolic hypertension. If systolic pressure is below 200, confirm within two months. If reading is 200 or more, refer for care within two weeks.

DIASTOLIC PRESSURE

Less than 85: normal. Recheck within two years.

85-89: high normal. Recheck within one year.

90-104: mild high blood pressure or hypertension. Confirm within two months. Whether or not treatment is indicated in this range is controversial, particularly when the numbers are between 90 and 94.

105-114: moderate hypertension. Refer for care within two weeks.

115 or higher: severe hypertension. Refer for immediate care.

At one time it was believed that by reducing blood pressure with medication we could also reduce heart attacks and strokes. But further studies demonstrated that, while reduced blood pressure yielded a reduced rate of strokes, the rate of heart attacks remained the same. Evidently, if the medication reduced pressure either too much or too little, the risk of heart attack remained present.

The latest studies recommend a reduction of 7 to 17 mmHg for people with mild to moderate hypertension. If she could achieve this reduction naturally, without medication, Marissa would not have to worry that she was reducing her blood pressure either too much, or too little.

How Should I Proceed?

If you already know you have high blood pressure and are on medication, you should not stop taking it. Instead, after consultation with your doctor, adopt the measures I recommend, and then, after a sufficient trial period — say a month or two — get a pressure reading that will indicate if the new steps you're taking are having an effect. It's quite likely that your pressure will be lower and you'll be able to reduce your medication.

If you have a "high normal" pressure reading, you're in a great position to profit from the help that natural medicine can offer. By adopting the suggestions below, you'll probably be able to lower your pressure naturally and avoid medication entirely.

While natural therapy can be very effective as a means of reducing and controlling hypertension, it does require a commitment to major lifestyle changes. While we don't know exactly what causes hypertension, we do know that it appears to be limited to developing nations. People in remote and non-industrial areas of the globe, such as the Solomon Islands and New Guinea, do not suffer from hypertension, even as they age. This suggests that hypertension may be a lifestyle disease, and must be treated accordingly, by adjusting various aspects of your everyday routines.

I told Marissa, as I tell all my patients with hypertension, that they must discontinue both smoking and drinking. If they are overweight, they must lose weight — even 5 to 10 pounds can make a significant difference. A diet high in fiber and low in saturated fats is also a key factor in blood pressure reduction, as are certain nutrients and supplements.

I gave Marissa my recommendations for natural therapy for hypertension, and then talked with her about exercise and stress reduction. I believe that high levels of stress are implicated in many of the medical ills of our society, and working women are particularly subject to stress, facing as they do the double challenge of running a household and performing at a highly competitive and stressful job.

Two months later, when Marissa returned to my office, she had lowered her blood pressure from 96 diastolic, a mild high, to 89 diastolic, a high normal reading, "And I want to bring it down to normal range," she said, beaming at me, highly pleased with herself.

I've noticed time and again that people who succeed in controlling a problem through natural therapy feel reinforced by their success, and the reinforcement in turn motivates them to further effort. In Marissa's case, she credited the drop in her blood pressure to dietary changes, and to stress reduction techniques.

"I used to have a steak and red wine whenever I took my clients out to dinner," she said, "and now I just order a salad or the vegetable plate or perhaps grilled fish. For the first time in my life, I'm as particular about what I eat as I am about what fuel to put into my car," she said. She was still working on stress reduction efforts, though she had made a good start by beginning an exercise routine. "I've been getting up half an hour earlier so I could work out or go for a jog — and now my husband's joined me, and it's doing both of us a lot of good."

I have many other patients with mild to moderate hypertension who, like Marissa, effectively control their blood pressure without the use of medication. I also have patients whose severe hypertension requires medication, but they too feel better and have been able to reduce the amount of medication needed through natural therapy. If you suffer from hypertension in any degree, or if there is a history of hypertension in your family and you want to prevent its onset, you will find the guidelines below helpful and effective.

If You Are Overweight, Lose Weight

You may say that's easier said than done, but you don't have to achieve your ideal weight to reduce blood pressure — even a small reduction will show significant results. So, if the prospect of losing fifty pounds is discouraging, try for a loss of 5 to 10 pounds as a start. In one study which tested various natural treatments for their effectiveness in reducing blood pressure, weight loss was the most effective!

Stop Smoking And Drinking

You already know that smoking causes cancer and heart disease. It also promotes hypertension, because nicotine stimulates the adrenal glands, which in turn increase blood pressure. Fewer people realize that alcohol is also linked to hypertension. Though there have been reports that "moderate" alcohol levels have a protective effect on the heart, I believe the definite risks of myocardial damage and hypertension far outweigh these possible benefits.

Since the negative effects associated with alcohol disappear when you stop drinking, I advise my patients with any degree of hypertension to discontinue all alcohol consumption.

Improve Your Nutritional Status

A diet high in fiber and low in saturated fat and cholesterol is of critical importance to patients with hypertension. A number of studies have linked saturated fat with increased blood pressure: when the saturated fat was decreased, or replaced with polyunsaturated fat, the blood pressure dropped accordingly. An ideal diet for hypertension would be a vegetarian diet, because it tends to be high in fiber, vitamin C, magnesium, calcium and potassium, and low in total fat, saturated fat, salt and cholesterol.

I don't unilaterally recommend a vegetarian diet to my patients — while many people thrive on a vegetarian diet, others find it leaves them feeling tired and rundown — I do advise them to adopt as many aspects of a vegetarian diet as possible. High fiber, so important to your overall good health, is essential to patients with hypertension. The emphasis here should not be on fiber supplements, but rather on fresh fruits, vegetables, legumes, and whole grain cereals. A high fiber cereal for breakfast, such as oat bran cereal, is a good way to increase your fiber intake.

Celery To The Rescue

Celery, which lowers blood pressure by relaxing the smooth muscles in the blood vessels, has been shown to lower blood pressure. Celery has a high sodium content, and you should not eat it if you are sodium sensitive. (See section "**What About Salt**," below.)

But for those who are not sensitive to salt, four stalks of celery daily will supply sufficient amounts of the active chemical to achieve its benefits. You may want to try celery daily for one week before a reading to see if it lowers your pressure. Don't overdose on celery, however, because it can be toxic in extremely large amounts.

Garlic For Hypertension

Garlic is also extremely effective in reducing blood pressure, and has been shown to reduce systolic pressure by 20 to 30 mmHg, and diastolic pressure by 10 to 20 mmHg. I tell my patients to enjoy garlic in food as often as possible. It must be fresh garlic, however, not the powdered or paste kind, and, as you need to take two or three cloves a day to get a therapeutic benefit, many people prefer to take the odor-free supplements available at health food stores.

Fish Oils And Blood Pressure

Fish oils and omega-3 fatty acid have also been shown to reduce blood pressure. Mackerel, salmon and tuna fish are all rich in omega-3 fatty acids. To insure a consistent consumption of omega-3 fatty acids I recommend Maxx EPA supplements to my patients.

What About Salt?

Until recently, salt was believed to raise blood pressure, and patients with hypertension were always told to eliminate salt from their diet. We now know that only about 30 to 40 percent of all people are sensitive to salt. To find out if you are salt sensitive, follow a salt-free diet for two weeks before your next blood pressure reading. If you've been abstaining from salt, on the other hand, try a moderate consumption of salt for two weeks before your next reading, and see if there's any difference.

If you are salt sensitive, you may also be getting an insufficient amount of potassium in your diet, which causes an increase in the volume of fluid and impairs the blood pressure mechanism. An interesting study showed that people were able to reduce their medications for hypertension by half, simply by consuming a diet rich in potassium. Vegetables and fresh fruits rich in potassium include potatoes, peas, peppers, eggplants, pears, squash, lima beans, tomatoes, and bananas. If you don't want to rely on food sources alone, you can also take a potassium supplement.

A Warning. . .

People with heart or kidney problems, whose bodies don't eliminate sodium efficiently, should always follow a salt-restricted diet.

For additional information on nutrition, see A HEALTHY WOMAN'S DAILY ROUTINE, page 19.

Nutritional Supplements For Hypertension

I recommend a number of supplements to my patients with hypertension, starting with calcium and magnesium. I mention them together because they work together in the body, and because low levels of both have been linked to high blood pressure. Studies have shown that supplements of calcium and magnesium are very effective for some patients, but have no effect on others. I suggest you take supplements of both for two months, and discontinue if there is no reduction in blood pressure.

Coenzyme Q-10, which is believed to improve the function of the blood vessel wall, is a supplement that's been extremely helpful for many people with cardiovascular disease, including people with hypertension. In one ten-week trial, hypertension patients taking Co Q-10 experienced a mean systolic and diastolic pressure reduction of 10.6 and 7.7 mmHg respectively, while those taking a placebo experienced no change.

Vitamin C also plays a role in regulating blood pressure, and recent studies have shown that, while it may have no impact on diastolic pressure, it definitely reduces systolic pressure readings.

Exercise And Hypertension

Exercise is tremendously beneficial to the cardiovascular system, because, in addition to its physiological effects, it works to reduce stress. One recent study showed the effects of exercise on people with moderate hypertension. These people, who were not taking medication for hypertension, exercised three or four times a week over a six month period, at which time their average systolic drop was 5 mmHg, and the average diastolic drop was 8 mmHg.

If you suffer from any degree of hypertension, you must make a commitment to exercise, even if it's only walking briskly for half an hour, three or four times a week. Review your exercise program with your doctor, and avoid exercises such as weight lifting, which causes a temporary — and drastic — increase in blood pressure.

Stress Control: Your Secret Weapon

Learning to control stress is a very important technique for lowering high blood pressure. One study, which focused on yoga and biofeedback in a controlled trial, showed a significant reduction in blood pressure using these stress control techniques.

I urge all my patients who suffer from hypertension to take stress control seriously and try to adopt techniques that will help them take a very important step in lowering their blood pressure. For further information, see STRESS CONTROL, page 321.

A Natural Treatment For Hypertension

An Important Warning. . .

If you are taking medication for hypertension, do not discontinue. Consult with your physician, adopt the changes recommended here and get a pressure reading two to three months later to see if your pressure is lowered and if you can reduce your medication. If your pressure is "high normal," adopt the recommendations below and you will probably be able to avoid the use of medication entirely.

- If you are overweight, lose weight. This change alone can sometimes lower your pressure into the normal range. Just five to ten pounds can make a difference.

- Lower your fat intake. See **Blueprint for Health**, page 21.

- Adopt as many relevant features of a vegetarian diet as possible including: more polyunsaturated fat, fiber, vitamin C, vitamin E, magnesium, calcium and potassium (see recommendations below for vitamin/mineral doses) and reduce total fat, saturated fat and cholesterol. Potassium-rich foods such as peas, peppers, eggplant and pears are especially helpful.

- Determine if you are salt sensitive. If sodium is affecting your blood pressure, eliminate it from your diet (see text).

- If you are salt sensitive and therefore must reduce sodium in your diet, take 100 mg. of potassium daily. (Potassium supplements will not interfere with medications.)

- Adopt a high fiber diet. Try oat bran cereal, or some other high fiber cereal, for breakfast. Increase your intake of fresh fruits and vegetables, whole grain cereals, breads and pastas. Do not take fiber supplements in connection with hypertension.

- Try eating three or four stalks of celery daily a week before a pressure reading to see if it helps. As celery contains a lot of sodium, don't do this if you are sodium-sensitive. (Don't eat celery in extremely large amounts as it can be toxic.)

- If you drink alcohol, stop. Eliminate alcohol from your diet.

In addition to your daily basic antioxidant vitamin/ mineral supplement, take:

- Calcium and magnesium. Take both supplements for a trial period of two months. Take 1200 mg. of calcium at bedtime and 250 mg. of magnesium 2 to 3 times daily. Follow this regime for two months and then check your pressure to see if the supplements have helped. If not, discontinue.
- Coenzyme Q-10: 30 mg. three times daily.
- Max EPA: 1000 mg. three times daily.
- Garlic: Increase consumption of garlic and other foods in the onion family. You can try garlic supplements that are available in health food stores. Take 1300 mg. in long-acting, odor-free capsules daily.
- Vitamin C: 1000 mg. daily.

Also

- Adopt an exercise program. Exercise for a half-hour, three to four times weekly. A brisk walk is excellent exercise.
- Adopt a stress control program. See STRESS CONTROL, page 321, for more information on how to do this.
- If you smoke, stop.

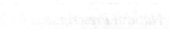

CHAPTER 22

Hypoglycemia

I have had a number of patients with hypoglycemia, or low blood sugar, over the years. Hypoglycemics are people who produce too much insulin in reaction to ingested sugar and, since insulin is a hormone that controls blood sugar levels, excessive insulin causes their sugar level to fall sharply. Symptoms of hypoglycemia include fatigue, headaches, anxiety, depression, dizziness, and late afternoon exhaustion.

Many of my patients had gone to other doctors who had dismissed their symptoms as psychosomatic. And yet, when these same people followed my nutritional program for hypoglycemia, they soon felt better than they had for months — or years.

There's been a good deal of controversy in the medical world about hypoglycemia. All doctors are familiar with the severe hypoglycemia experienced on occasion by diabetics and people with other serious conditions, yet many doctors ignore, and refuse to acknowledge, the low level, borderline hypoglycemia caused by eating too much sugar and refined carbohydrates.

Consequently, many people with hypoglycemia continue to suffer needlessly — and aggravate their condition each time they eat a sugar snack to boost their flagging energy, thus releasing insulin which sends their sugar level into a nosedive.

Kimberly, a college junior, had been caught up in this vicious cycle, and as a result was having trouble keeping up with her courses.

"I'm so tired all the time, especially in the afternoon," she told me, "and in fact, a couple of times I have fallen asleep in class — which is not the way to endear yourself to your professors. And I'm just tired all the time, and headachy. I don't know what's wrong with me. . . I used to get straight A's in school, but the way things are going this year I might as well drop out and go back home."

Kimberly, as it turned out, had lived at home for her first two years at college, and had recently transferred to a college in New York City so she could study Japanese, which would be useful in her family's import-export business. She was a short, pretty girl with an attractive smile, but she was slightly overweight for her small frame, and her skin was pale, with a somewhat pasty quality.

Her problems had started soon after she left home. Now she felt anxious and depressed much of the time, and she had sometimes wondered if all her problems were in her mind — if they were due to homesickness.

During her examination, Kimberly told me her daily diet had undergone a drastic change when she had left home. Now she lived in a dormitory and grabbed a bite to eat whenever she could — usually a donut or muffin for breakfast, pizza for dinner, and whatever she could manage to snag in between. She usually took a candy bar along, she said, in case she didn't have time for a proper lunch. Kimberly had never heard of hypoglycemia, and was surprised when I told her she had low blood sugar — because of too much sugar in her diet.

Many of my patients with hypoglycemia have been taken aback to discover that the sugar they eat is to blame for their low blood sugar levels, and yet the mechanics of it are fairly simple. As soon as the sugar you eat reaches your blood — which happens within seconds after you eat it — the pancreas releases insulin, the hormone used to regulate blood sugar levels.

If you don't regularly eat too much sugar and have no tendency to hypoglycemia, your body has no trouble maintaining a proper sugar balance. But if you have some trouble in handling an excessive amount of sugar, the pancreas overacts and floods your body with insulin, and your sugar levels plummet.

That's not all. The adrenal glands, alerted that something is wrong, start releasing antistress hormones, which, in turn, release the sugar stored in the liver for emergencies. Of course, over a period of time all this activity is wearing on the system, and in the meantime you experience weakness, fatigue, dizziness, headaches, and anxiety.

Her symptoms of depression and anxiety, I told Kimberly, were not in her mind, but in her brain. The brain is more dependent on blood sugar, or glucose, than any other organ, and it requires a constant supply to function properly. Low blood sugar levels impact the functioning of the brain, and result in a lack of mental alertness, mood swings, headaches, and the other symptoms common to people who have difficulty in handling refined sugar.

Kimberly, who had year-end exams coming up, was hoping that I would give her some medication to boost her energy. But Kimberly didn't need medication, she needed to get her metabolic system back into balance. I told Kimberly to try my nutritional program for hypoglycemia which has helped so many of my patients regain a level of energy and a feeling of well-being they had forgotten.

The first step of the program, is — no surprise here — eliminating all sugar from the diet. This means doing some detective work, because much of the sugar we eat is in prepared foods and refined carbohydrates. Americans consume eighty pounds of sugar a year, or about thirty teaspoons a day, and much of it is hidden in prepared foods such as canned soups, frozen meals, and even salad dressings. And of course simple carbohydrates such as white flour, white rice and potatoes are also quickly converted into sugar.

I told Kimberly that fiber and complex carbohydrates, both of which help to stabilize blood sugar, should become a mainstay of her diet. The most natural the form of food, the better. Whole grain bread is better than white bread, an apple better than apple juice. Protein, which stimulates less of an insulin response, is also important to someone with hypoglycemia, and should be eaten at each meal.

I warned Kimberly that she should stop skipping meals, because regular food intake keeps blood sugar stable. If she did have to skip a meal on occasion, I suggested she drink a glass of skim milk or eat a piece of fruit to tide her over. In fact, many of my patients with hypoglycemia eat a mid-morning and mid-afternoon snack to keep their blood sugar on an even keel.

Finally, I recommended that she take chromium, a trace mineral utilized to control insulin production, which has proven to be near miraculous in controlling blood sugar and reducing sugar cravings.

I was pleased but not surprised when, two weeks later, Kimberly called to report that the simple program I had given her had been more effective than she could have imagined.

"Almost miraculous!" she said, adding that the fatigue, the mood swings, the depression were all gone. "And, as an added bonus, I've lost five pounds of the weight I'd gained this term."

I'm convinced that sugar has negative physiological effects in the long run, even for people who don't have hypoglycemia. I recommend that all my patients reduce or eliminate sugar from their diet. If you believe you have hypoglycemia, or merely wish to feel a sense of renewed energy, I recommend the following program.

Eliminate Sugar From Your Diet

When you eliminate sugar, it's not enough to hide the sugar bowl and stay away from sugar-filled products, such as candy, cookies and cakes, ice cream, sodas, honey and other sweetened foods. You must learn to read the labels of canned and frozen products to determine how much sugar they actually contain.

Ingredients on a label are listed in descending order by amount, so if sugar is second or third on the list you can assume the product contains a good deal of sugar. Unfortunately, it's not that cut-and-dried, because many sugar additives are listed under different names, so you must identify them and then add them up together to determine how much sugar the product actually contains!

Sugar Additives Most Commonly Listed On Food Labels	
Corn Syrup	Maple
Fructose	Molasses
Glucose	Sorghum
Lactose	Sucrose
Maltose	Syrup

Most people realize that jams, or canned fruit and juice probably contain added sugar, but many of my patients were surprised to discover that products such as canned soup. spaghetti sauce and peanut butter are also loaded with sugar. Study the labels, and choose products without sugar additives.

Avoid Simple Carbohydrates

Since simple carbohydrates are converted very quickly into sugar, it's best to stick to fiber and complex carbohydrates, which help to stabilize blood sugar levels. Instead of baked products made with white flour, buy bread made with whole grains. Use brown rice instead of white rice, an apple instead of apple juice. Whole grain products and legumes should make up a large part of your diet.

Eat Regular Meals At Regular Times

If you have hypoglycemia and need to stabilize your blood sugar, it is essential that you eat your meals at regular times. Don't skip breakfast or lunch, don't have a late breakfast or a late lunch or dinner. Try to eat your meals at regular intervals, at the same time each day.

Some doctors believe that as many as six to eight small meals throughout the day are better for hypoglycemics than the standard three. Since this is too inconvenient for most people, however, I recommend that you eat a mid-morning and a mid-afternoon snack in addition to your regular meals, and another light snack just before going to bed. A piece of fruit, or whole wheat toast with fruit butter, whole wheat crackers, popcorn and rice cakes all make appropriate snacks — just make sure they're free of sugar additives!

Improve Your Nutritional Status

Protein produces less of an insulin response than carbohydrates, and should be included with each meal. An egg-white omelet is a good source of protein for breakfast. For lunch and dinner, I suggest fish, chicken, or turkey. If you don't have time for a cooked meal, water-packed tuna and water-packed sardines provide a good supply of protein.

It is also essential that you eat a nutritious diet and take supplements when appropriate to fulfill your nutritional needs. Refer to **A HEALTHY WOMAN'S DAILY ROUTINE**, page 19, for nutritional guidelines.

Avoid Alcohol, Smoking And Caffeine

Avoid alcohol, smoking and caffeine, which cause drastic fluctuations in blood sugar levels and tend to be addictive for hypoglycemic patients. While one cup of coffee in the morning is acceptable, I tell my patients that they should eat something beforehand, and that they should limit themselves to that one cup. Don't drink coffee or caffeinated drinks later in the day, and check over-the-counter medications for caffeine.

I also recommend that my patients stay away from artificial sweeteners, partially because of associated health problems, but mostly because they promote continued sweet cravings. Many of my patients who had a real sweet tooth were surprised to discover their sugar cravings diminished a few weeks after they gave up sugar. Artificial sweeteners, on the other hand, tend to prolong and reinforce the sugar craving.

The Miracle Supplement For Hypoglycemia

Chromium, a trace mineral utilized by the body for the proper function of insulin, is deficient from the daily diet of most Americans. My patients who took chromium supplements three times a day before meals were amazed at its effectiveness in controlling their sweet cravings and keeping up their energy levels between meals.

A Natural Treatment For Hypoglycemia

- Eliminate sugar from the diet. That means no cakes, candies, cookies, ice cream, sweetened cereal, canned fruit, frozen desserts, etc. In addition, you must learn to read food labels to find hidden sources of sugar. See above for how to assess a food label.

- Avoid simple carbohydrates and refined and processed foods such as instant rice and instant potatoes, white flour, soft drinks, alcohol, etc.

- Eat a diet high in complex carbohydrates and fiber, both of which help to stabilize blood sugar. Try to stick to the most natural, unprocessed form of a food.

- Eat regular meals at regular times. Don't skip meals. Don't eat late meals.
- Eliminate alcohol and smoking.
- Limit your caffeine intake to one caffeinated beverage — coffee or tea — daily. Watch out for caffeinated soft drinks and over-the-counter drugs that contain caffeine.
- Eliminate the use of artificial sweeteners.

In addition to your daily basic antioxidant vitamin/mineral, take:

- Chromium: the trivalent form, in dosages of 100 micrograms three times a day before meals.

CHAPTER 23

Insomnia

Insomnia is a widespread problem in our society. It's estimated that, on any given night, one out of three people will have trouble going to sleep, or will wake up and toss and turn in the small hours. The occasional sleepless night is no cause for concern, though it may leave you feeling tired and out of sorts the next day. But when a pattern of insomnia sets in, and you become sleep-deprived over a long period of time, your health may become impaired, while your ability to function at your best is severely curtailed.

Many of my patients have had trouble with insomnia. Sometimes it's because they are facing a particularly stressful situation or personal crisis. Sometimes it's due to hormonal changes such as those that occur before a period or due to menopause. But much more often it's because their evening routine promotes sleeplessness: it's difficult to fall asleep if you feel mentally or physically stimulated. If you do demanding work too late into the evening, or exercise too late, or eat too much of the wrong thing, or drink alcohol or caffeine, you may well experience problems falling asleep.

Such was the case with Megan, an old-time patient who came in for a routine checkup one day last Spring. Megan, a mother of two who went back to work for a sports chain store after her divorce some years ago, told me she felt well enough. But she looked tense, pale, and the deep dark circles beneath her eyes were very noticeable in spite of her attempts to cover them with makeup.

"The fact is that I'm desperate for sleep," she admitted. "Oh, I fall asleep soon enough when I turn out the light — I'm so tired that I'm out cold the minute I close my eyes. But then I wake up — at two, or three o'clock in the morning — and think about all the things I need to do the next day, or next week, or next year. Sometimes I turn the light on and read, other times I get a glass of milk. Either way I can't go back to sleep for hours. I'm exhausted when the alarm goes off, and need two or three cups of coffee before I can really wake up."

Megan, as it turned out, would also drink a cup or two of coffee at lunch, in addition to a couple of caffeinated sodas in the afternoon: the equivalent of six or more cups of caffeine a day. With that much caffeine in her system, insomnia was a given. I recommended that she cut back to one cup of coffee a day.

I also recommended that she deal with her anxiety. Like other single working mothers, Megan had a long list of responsibilities, and was always nervous that something important would fall by the wayside. I suggested that she could reduce her nighttime anxieties by setting aside a specific time during the day — during her commute to work, maybe — for activity planning.

I also suggested that the old-fashioned glass of milk at bedtime might prove helpful. Milk is rich in the amino acid tryptophan, which is helpful in naturally inducing sleep.

But when Megan asked me about sleeping pills, I told her I was absolutely opposed to their use.

The Sleeping Pill Trap

When people start taking sleeping pills, they think their insomnia problems are over. But within a few weeks the effect of the pills starts to wear off, and they wake up during the night. They need ever greater amounts of sleeping pills to do the job, and then start to feel the negative side effects.

Sleeping pills interfere with normal sleep, and actually decrease REM, or rapid-eye-movement sleep — the most restful phase of sleep during which brain cells are restored. The loss of REM sleep promotes irritability, depression and anxiety, and decreases memory and concentration levels.

A recent study showed that some users of sleeping pills suffered alarming side effects such as unsteady gait, dizziness, and depression.

Valerie, a woman who had been taking sleeping pills for a year, once came to see me, desperate for help. Valerie, whose picture appeared occasionally in the society pages, was an attractive, fashionable woman in her mid-fifties, married to the C.E.O. of a major corporation. She had two children who were doing well in their professions. She had a large apartment in the city and a weekend getaway at the seashore.

Unlike Megan, Valerie had little to worry about. And yet Valerie was desperate for sleep. The sleeping pills she had been taking for so long had lost their effectiveness, and Valerie would get up late after a sleepless night, drink endless cups of coffee, have lunch, and then, exhausted, come home and take an afternoon nap. Since the pills no longer worked, she had started having a drink or two in the evening, in addition to wine with dinner — but even the alcohol didn't seem to help.

As Valerie talked, her face remained calm and composed and her soft voice uninflected, and yet I sensed an emotional disturbance beneath the surface calm. Insomnia has long been associated with depression, and over half the cases of insomnia have a psychological cause. I felt fairly certain this was the case with Valerie and, when I asked her if anything was troubling her, she replied, still in that soft voice, yes, everything was troubling her. Her children had grown, her husband had grown distant, and her days were empty. She dreaded the beginning of each day.

I told Valerie that I thought she would benefit from seeing a psychologist and, after a minute's hesitation, she agreed. She sounded relieved, I thought. But first of all, I told her, she should give up sleeping pills, alcohol, and caffeine. The mixture of sleeping pills and alcohol is potentially deadly, even in small doses, and caffeine, which is an addictive substance, is a cause of insomnia.

I warned Valerie that it might take up to five weeks for the sleeping pills to be cleaned out of her system. In the meantime, however, she could start following some of the techniques I have found to be effective against insomnia.

Medication Alert. . .

In addition to coffee, there are a number of medications that can cause sleepless nights. There are cold medications that contain phenylpropanolamine, there are blood pressure medications and appetite suppressants, there's Inderal and other beta blockers, and Dilantin for the prevention of seizures. If you suffer from insomnia and believe it might be due to a prescription medication, you should obviously discuss it with your doctor.

Low Blood Sugar And Insomnia

Low blood sugar, or hypoglycemia, can also cause people to wake in the middle of the night, when their blood sugar drops. I tell my patients with low blood sugar that they should eat a light snack before bedtime, such as a piece of fruit or some crackers — without sugar, of course. If you suffer from fatigue in the morning, and also feel tired and irritable around four o'clock in the afternoon, you might have low blood sugar. See HYPOGLYCEMIA, page 243.

Good Sleep Habits

One of the most effective ways of combating insomnia is to develop good sleeping habits, the most important one being the habit of going to bed at the same time each night. It's important for the body to establish its own sleeping rhythm. If you stay up late and sleep in late on the weekend, you may have trouble sleeping soundly on Monday night, no matter how tired you are.

Similarly, if you take a nap during the day, you will sleep less soundly at night. I suggest that you avoid naps during the day unless you are sick or are scheduled to work or travel during the night.

Finally, allow your mind and your body to wind down for a couple of hours before you go to bed. Read, or watch television, or listen to music, or take a warm bath. Avoid strenuous exercise, and avoid tension-filled activities. If you have insomnia, it's really not a good idea to sit down one hour before bedtime to balance out a checkbook or do your taxes.

Both Megan and Valerie had developed poor sleeping habits and, to my surprise, it was Valerie, with the more serious problem, who was the first one to turn herself around. She rose to the challenge and went cold turkey on sleeping pills, alcohol, and caffeine. She joined a gym and signed up for a daily exercise routine. She developed the habit of drinking a glass of skim milk and taking a calcium supplement at night. And she started going to the psychologist I'd recommended for help in getting through what she referred to as her mid-life crisis.

"I go to bed early and sleep through the night," she told me three months later. She had started doing volunteer work for a local kitchen, and found she had organizational skills she had never suspected. "It's much easier to sleep well when you are really tired," Valerie said.

Megan, on the other hand, who, being a working mother, was always tired, not to say exhausted, had developed insomnia in spite of it. She too gave up all caffeine for awhile. She found that if she wrote down her worries and plans during the day, they were less apt to wake her up at night. She too started taking calcium before going to bed.

But she still had occasional problems with insomnia until she started using valerian, an herb which depresses the central nervous system and relaxes smooth muscle tissue. Valerian has been used for years as a sedative, and promotes healthful sleep without any of the drugged aftereffects of a sleeping pill.

Another helpful herb against insomnia is passionflower, a sedative and analgesic herb which can be made into a tea, and is available at the health food stores.

What About Melatonin?

Many of my patients ask about the use of melatonin for insomnia and I recommend it with certain caveats. When melatonin first became popular for sleeping problems, many people began to take it routinely. But research has now shown that this can cause problems, as a regular dose can cause the body to "forget" how to produce its own melatonin. Thus the user becomes the "addict" and melatonin supplementation becomes mandatory.

To avoid this, I recommend using melatonin only for occasional insomnia and not on a regular basis. If you want to try melatonin, get the sublingual tablets (the ones that dissolve under your tongue) as they seem to work best.

Basic Techniques Against Insomnia Which Have Proved Effective For Many Of My Patients.

Eliminate Stimulants

Give up coffee and caffeinated drinks, or cut back to no more than one cup of coffee a day. Check with your doctor to determine if any of your prescription medications contain stimulants, and check the label on your over-the-counter medications for stimulants than can keep you awake.

Check For Low Blood Sugar

If you wake up tired in the morning, and also feel a sharp drop of energy in the afternoon, you may be suffering from low blood sugar, or hypoglycemia. See HYPOGLYCEMIA (page 243) for sugges-

tions on how to deal with this problem. To keep from waking in the night when your blood sugar drops, eat a snack or have a glass of skim milk just before bedtime.

Develop Good Sleeping Habits

The most important thing you can do to banish insomnia is to develop the habit of going to bed at the same time each night. Allow your body and mind to relax two hours before bedtime. One of my patients with insomnia found it helpful to dim the overhead lights in her room one hour before going to sleep.

Avoid naps, or sleeping in late on weekends. A regular routine will allow your body to develop and get used to a regular sleep/wake rhythm.

Work On Relaxation Techniques

Physical exercise promotes a sense of well-being and relaxation, and should be a part of your regular daily routine. However, since the initial effect of exercise is stimulating, do it in the morning, or at that low ebb in the afternoon when you need a pick-up. Avoid exercising just before bedtime, when it's counterproductive.

For people who need additional help to relax, there are books on relaxation techniques, and tapes on self-hypnosis. Just counting sheep has been effective for some of my patients, while others pretend they are lying on a warm Caribbean beach, breathing in and out to the rhythm of the waves. I recommend Herbert Benson's *Relaxation Response* for detailed information on various relaxation techniques.

Try Nutritional And Herbal Supplements

A glass of warm milk at bedtime will help to make you sleepy, because it contains L-tryptophan, an amino acid that induces sleep. Turkey and tuna are also good natural sources of L-tryptophan. L-tryptophan was available as a supplement until a few years ago, when a contaminated batch prompted the government to ban it from the market. I think that someday L-tryptophan will become available again in supplement form, but until it does use the natural form found in foods.

Milk also contains calcium, of course, which promotes relaxation. Many of my patients with insomnia like to take a calcium supplement at bedtime.

Valerian and passionflower are natural herbs that have been used for many years to promote sleep and reduce anxiety. They have no problematic side effects, and I have patients who swear by them.

A Natural Treatment For Insomnia

- Check your medications. Some common medications can cause insomnia.
- Eliminate caffeine, including all caffeinated beverages — don't forget colas and other soft drinks — as well as chocolate.

You can try one caffeinated beverage in the morning but nothing more.

- Stop smoking, or at least don't have a cigarette within a few hours of bedtime as it's a stimulant.

- Avoid stimulation at bedtime, including any work or reading that is likely to produce anxiety.

- Don't take naps even if you're tired at a certain point in the day. Try to exercise at this time instead.

- Develop regular sleep habits, going to bed and getting up at virtually the same time every day.

- Until and unless the natural supplement L-tryptophan comes onto the market again, rely on natural sources of it, including turkey and tuna or even a glass of milk before bed.

- Try the herb valerian: take 2 capsules one hour before bedtime.

- Take a cup of passionflower tea before bedtime.

- Get regular daily exercise, avoiding exercise close to bedtime.

- Try relaxation techniques at bedtime.

In addition to your daily basic antioxidant vitamin/ mineral supplement, take:

- Calcium: 1200 mg. at bedtime.

An Update On A New Supplement For Sleep

Another supplement that can be helpful in promoting sleep is ornithine. I've never used ornithine but the latest research on it is encouraging. Some researchers have found it to be as effective as tryptophan in promoting sleep. As it's quite without side effects and safe, you might give it a try. It's available in 500 mg. capsules and you take two the first night and four on subsequent nights for a week. If no results, discontinue.

CHAPTER 24

Menopause

Barbara was my first patient of the day. I had been seeing her off and on for about ten years and was familiar with her medical history as well as her personality. She was an office manager in a large law firm and I'm sure she was terrific at her job. She had an air of no-nonsense efficiency about her and was always very eager to get in to see me and get out as quickly as possible. I was surprised, therefore, to see her sitting in front of me looking tired and slightly disheveled.

"Dr. Giller, I hope you can help me. I've had the worst few months. I'm not sleeping well. I'm feeling much more tired than usual. Of course, that could simply be because I'm not sleeping." Barbara managed a weak smile.

"And I'm getting weird symptoms: my fingers tingle sometimes. My colleagues have told me —

those that dare — that I'm really irritable lately. And sometimes I find I just can't focus; I'm sitting at my desk and for a moment or two I have no idea what I'm supposed to be doing. I'm getting a little frightened by all this and I wonder if I could have some sort of auto-immune disease or something."

At a vital and attractive forty six, it's no wonder that Barbara never thought she could be menopausal. Indeed, she was somewhat young to be showing early signs of menopause but she was truly relieved when I explained that was what was causing her symptoms.

Barbara, like many women, thought menopause just happened out of the blue like a first period: you reached a certain age and your periods stopped and then you were in menopause and you got symptoms. She was amazed to learn that the symptoms can begin before the actual menopause. And she was also pleased to learn that many of her symptoms could be readily treated with natural treatments.

Menopause Today

I have been very happy to see so much information on menopause getting out to the public these days. In the past, menopause was too often a deep, dark secret and many of my women patients were terribly confused about what to expect and how to cope with the changes that occur at midlife.

Nonetheless, there's still lots of misinformation to sort out if you are a woman who's trying to make sense of what this inevitable marker will mean to you. Menopause used to be a virtual mystery; before the 1900's most women died around the age of fifty, a few years before the average onset of menopause. As women lived longer, there were doctors who denied that menopause was anything but a psychological problem. Tranquilizers were thought to be the solution.

Today, most women are familiar with the well-known symptoms of menopause: hot flashes, headaches, sleep disturbances, vaginal dryness and changes in sexual function and desire. But there are other, long-term results of menopause that are the source of today's controversy.

At the heart of the controversy is whether menopause and its physical changes should be viewed as a natural event to be endured (or simply ignored by the many women who experience few symptoms), or whether it is an evolutionary mistake that can be corrected by the use of drugs.

The Stages Of Menopause

Menopause doesn't happen overnight: on Monday you're your usual self and on Tuesday you don't get an expected period and you're therefore in menopause. Indeed, it's important to understand that the whole event of menopause is actually three stages in a woman's life:

Perimenopause is the first stage of menopause. It usually begins around the mid-forties although women will vary widely in their biological clocks. In perimenopause, the amount of estrogen produced by your ovaries begins to decline. Your periods will gradually become irregular over the next decade and the amount of menstrual flow will vary: sometimes it will be very light while at other times it will be copious. It is at this stage of the "change" — perimenopause — that many women will be troubled by symptoms, many of which are caused by fluctuating hormone levels. Some women will have many symptoms; others will have none.

Menopause, the next stage, actually occurs when your estrogen levels drop so low that you no longer have a period. This is the actual menopause — from the Greek that means "monthly" and "cease." Actual menopause lasts for one year, from your last period through the twelve months that follow.

Postmenopause, the last stage, will probably account for the most years of your life. It is the time when you no longer menstruate. Many women live longer as postmenopausal women than as fertile, menstruating ones.

> **Menopause refers to the actual cessation of menstrual periods but for many women the symptoms of menopause occur during perimenopause — the year or two or three — before actual menopause. This is confusing to many women because they sometimes begin to suffer vague symptoms before menopause and can't understand what's happening to their bodies. If you are suffering the vague symptoms described in this section and are between the ages of 40 and 50, (although women can, rarely, experience a menopause before the age of 40), visit your gynecologist to see if your symptoms could be related to menopause.**

Signs Of Menopause

The first sign of menopause for most women is irregular periods. The cycle may shorten or lengthen; the menstrual flow may increase or decrease. A woman can be fertile even if she's been without a period for a year. After a woman experiences irregular periods for a year to five years, menstruation will stop.

A year to a year and a half before a woman's periods end, she may experience hot flashes, during which her temperature will rise and fall as much as 9 degrees. These flashes may be accompanied by sweating, heart palpitations, nausea, and, not surprisingly, anxiety.

Hot flashes can contribute to insomnia; some women complain of waking frequently and having to change damp bedclothes. And some women also notice irritability, headaches, short-term memory loss, lack of sexual desire, and inability to concentrate. Some of these symptoms are not due to estrogen loss, but are simply a result of hot flashes and lack of adequate sleep.

Estrogen And Menopause

When you realize that more than three hundred types of tissues throughout the body have receptors for estrogen — which is to say that they're affected in some way by the hormone — it's not surprising that its decrease would cause physical changes.

Estrogen affects the genital organs (vagina, vulva, and uterus), the urinary organs (bladder and urethra), breasts, skin, hair, mucous membranes, bones, heart and blood vessels, pelvic muscles, and the brain.

It's the loss of estrogen to these organs that causes the ultimate changes of menopause, including dry skin and hair, incontinence and susceptibility to urinary tract infections, vaginal dryness, and, most important, the diseases osteoporosis and heart disease. These diseases are at the center of the controversy concerning menopause: because estrogen plays a role in preventing these diseases, should you replace the estrogen lost at the time of menopause with a synthetic version?

Not all women suffer the symptoms and diseases I've mentioned above. Many women sail through menopause with minimal discomfort. Some ten percent of women have absolutely no symptoms at all except for the end of their menstrual periods. A few women never have a hot flash, some experience one or two hot flashes a month, and others have several an hour. Just as some women experience debilitating symptoms of PMS while others are symptom free in relation to their menstrual cycle, so it is with menopause. Don't expect to have symptoms; you may be one of the lucky ones who have none at all.

Estrogen Replacement Therapy

Estrogen replacement therapy, or ERT, and whether or not to take it, is an option that women facing menopause will have to consider carefully. You should not rely on anyone, *including your doctor,* to make this decision for you. There are too many variables that affect your best course of action, and you alone can decide. Here are some of the factors to consider:

Benefits

- Prevents osteoporosis.
- Prevents heart attacks and strokes.
- Prevents hot flashes.
- Improves energy and mood.
- Eliminates insomnia.
- Prevents vaginal atrophy.
- Prevents weakening to pelvic muscles.
- Possible prevention or delay of Alzheimer's disease.

Risks

- Possible increase of endometrial cancer.
- Possible increased risk of breast cancer.
- Blood clots or hypertension.
- Gallstones.
- PMS-type symptoms including breast pain and tenderness.
- Frequent medical monitoring involving increased costs and potential for surgical procedures.

Reviewing these benefits and risks will help you decide on the wisdom of ERT for you. For example, if you have a family history of breast cancer or endometrial cancer, these factors argue against ERT in your case. But a strong family history of osteoporosis might incline you toward ERT. All of the facts concerning your background should be weighed and discussed with your doctor.

> Many women have doubts about using hormones in menopause: only 30 percent of women who are given prescriptions for hormone therapy ever fill them. There are still too many unanswered questions about hormone therapy to make blanket statements about who should and should not use it. You must be your own advocate on this matter. Read as much as you can and discuss your options with your doctor.

Remember that the decision concerning ERT need not be forever. Some women take ERT for a year or two or three to get them through a highly symptomatic time of their menopause and then discontinue it.

Whatever you decide concerning ERT, there are natural means you can employ to minimize the discomforts of menopause. I advise many of my women patients, who are wary of using hormones, to try natural remedies first. For many women, a natural approach will help them control menopausal symptoms without ever using hormones.

Symptoms Of Menopause

Hot flashes are, for some women, the most troublesome symptom of menopause. They cause insomnia, resulting in irritability, and they can be uncomfortable and embarrassing. In my experience with my patients, drops in blood sugar can be the single most common precipitating cause of hot flashes. Once the blood sugar is controlled, the incidence of hot flashes diminishes.

In fact, by following the suggestions outlined in HYPOGLYCEMIA (page 243), particularly eliminating sugar, reducing caffeine, eating meals at regular times, eating protein at lunch and dinner, and taking the supplement chromium, many women have told me that their hot flashes were dramatically relieved.

Soy, The Miracle Bean

There are certain foods that can reduce menopausal symptoms. These foods, including soy flour, tofu, and other soy foods, as well as linseed oil, contain substances called phytoestrogens that can help compensate for the body's loss of estrogen at menopause. The plant estrogens in soy, called isoflavones, bear so strong a resemblance to the human hormone that they seem to fill in when a woman's own levels start to dip.

Interestingly, in some societies, half of the dietary intake includes foods that contain phytoestrogens; our typical diet contains less than 10 percent. Asian women, who eat a diet high in soy, rarely suffer from hot flashes or sleep disturbances; indeed, there's not even a word for hot flash in Japanese.

Researchers are just beginning to realize how helpful soy can be in combating menopausal symptoms. Indeed, from a health standpoint, soy can be seen as the miracle bean. In one study of healthy menopausal women who increased their intake of soy products or soy-containing foods for a period of six weeks, significant improvement was seen in the results of vaginal smears following the increased phytoestrogen consumption.

What is particularly exciting about the use of phytoestrogens to combat menopausal symptoms is that the effect of phytoestrogens on the body is without health risks. The use of both natural and synthetic estrogens increase the risk of cancer, gall-bladder disease as well as strokes. But phytoestrogens have not been associated with any of these negative side effects.

Moreover, soy products have other health benefits that make them particularly beneficial for women in the menopausal years. Studies have shown that as little as 25 grams of soy protein a day can lower cholesterol in people with high cholesterol.

A recent study published in *The New England Journal of Medicine* reported that an average daily consumption of 47 grams of soy lowered total cholesterol, low-density lipoprotein (LDL), and triglycerides. High-density lipoprotein (HDL), the so-called good cholesterol, went up a little, though this rise was not significant.

If that weren't enough, the components in soy protein may help prevent bone loss. For menopausal women who are facing the possibility of osteoporosis, this is excellent news.

And finally, soy products have been shown to help prevent a variety of cancers.

I recommend that all my women patients who are entering the perimenopausal years add soy to their diets. I think it's the simplest and best way to maintain long-term good health while avoiding menopausal symptoms.

Common forms of soy protein include tofu, soy milk, tempeh (a combination of fermented soybeans and grain), soy flour (used in baking), and soy protein powders, which come in a variety of flavors and can be mixed with water or juice.

Soy Shake

For a tasty breakfast drink or an afternoon pick-me-up, a soy shake is a great alternative to tea or coffee. The critical ingredient is soy protein powder which you can find at your health food store. Soy protein powder is an especially good way to get your soy because you can mix it into pancakes, meatloaves, soups or other foods.

Try this shake: Put about 6 oz. of orange juice in a blender. Add two or three cubes of ice and 2 heaping tablespoons of soy protein powder. Blend until foamy.

Another delicious shake can be made using a whole banana (you can cut it into chunks and freeze it first), 6 oz. of skim milk, a drizzle of honey and 2 heaping tablespoons of soy powder. Blend until foamy. Try using fresh or frozen berries in place of the banana.

Nutritional Supplements For Menopause

The mineral boron has proved very helpful for my menopausal patients. Boron naturally elevates estrogen levels and I originally recommended it to some patients to help fight osteoporosis. Many women told me that it had an immediate beneficial effect on their hot flashes.

Vitamin E has been helpful for many women who suffer from hot flashes and sometimes, when supplemented with vitamin C, it completely eliminates the symptom. Vitamin E is also useful because it decreases the tendency of blood platelets to clump together in menopausal women, which can contribute to heart attacks and strokes.

Many women complain of anxiety, irritability, and depression during menopause. As I've mentioned, these symptoms can be exacerbated by loss of sleep. Calcium supplementation generally has worked for all my patients, including menopausal patients, in helping them get to sleep and stay asleep. The mineral magnesium can also be helpful in relieving these symptoms.

Osteoporosis, which should be a concern for all women, becomes a pressing issue during menopause, when the estrogen supply diminishes and promotes increased bone loss. The most critical steps to take are to increase your calcium intake, in the form of foods and supplements, and to exercise. For more information, see OSTEOPOROSIS, page 303.

Heart disease also becomes a threat in the menopausal years. Prior to menopause, estrogen plays a protective role in relation to heart disease, but as estrogen production diminishes, the risk of heart disease increases. Ten years after menopause, a woman has nearly the same risk as a man of dying of heart disease. The major cause of this increased risk is a rise in the LDL ("bad") cholesterol and a lowering of the protective HDL cholesterol resulting in vulnerability to atherosclerosis.

In addition, the lack of estrogen causes the blood vessels to become less flexible, so blood clots can form more readily. Improved diet, exercise, and the use of supplements can all be helpful in preventing heart disease. For more detailed information, see **ATHEROSCLEROSIS**, page 83.

There is also an herb that can be helpful in relieving menopausal symptoms, including hot flashes and depression. Dong quai (*Angelica sinesis*) has been proven to affect estrogen activity, and many women find it beneficial.

Many of my women patients have never heard of black cohosh but, in fact, it is one of the most thoroughly studied and effective natural approaches to menopausal symptoms. Black cohosh (*Cirmcifuga racemosa*) is a perenniel plant, the underground stem of which is used to create a treatment that is remarkably effective in relieving not only hot flashes, but also depression and vaginal atrophy.

A standardized version of black cohosh is available under the name Remifemin and is available at your health food store. It has proven remarkably effective in many studies in giving women relief from symptoms that have been troubling them.

Menopause And Exercise

One of the most critical steps you can take to reduce the symptoms of menopause is to exercise. Countless studies have demonstrated that regular exercise can benefit menopausal women by fighting depression and anxiety, strengthening bone mass and lessening the risk of osteoporosis, reducing the risk of atherosclerosis, and improving one's overall quality of life. I strongly recommend that all menopausal women adopt an exercise program.

Many women find that walking is a form of exercise they can easily fit into their lifestyle and do on a year-round basis. Jane, one of my patients who was suffering from a troubling host of menopausal symptoms, including hot flashes, severe fatigue, irritability and inability to concentrate, told me that the single best recommendation I made to her was to exercise. While she's also taking some of the nutritional supplements I recommend, she feels that it's the exercise that's given her the greatest relief from her symptoms. She walks two miles at least four times a week with a friend. She says the conversation and companionship are as important to her as the actual exercise but she's noticed that her fatigue and hot flashes have been greatly reduced.

There are a number of excellent books available on walking programs that will inspire you. Of course other forms of exercise, such as swimming, aerobic classes, cycling, and dance are good choices, too. But exercise must be done regularly if it's to be of benefit. I suggest that you exercise for a half-hour five times a week.

Smoking: More Bad News

In addition to the myriad problems associated with cigarettes, smoking encourages an early menopause. Women who smoke experience menopause four to five years earlier than women who do not smoke. Smoking also increases your risk of many of the symptoms of menopause, including osteoporosis and heart disease.

A Natural Treatment For Menopause

- Discuss the advisability of estrogen replacement therapy with your doctor. See text for a full discussion of this.

- Control blood sugar levels in an effort to reduce hot flashes. See HYPOGLYCEMIA, page 243.

- Increase your intake of soy-containing foods, including tofu and soy flour, as well as linseed oil (which is available in capsule form in health food stores) in the amount of 500 mg. three times a day. Soy protein powder is a good and convenient source of soy.

- Reduce your risk of developing osteoporosis. See OSTEOPOROSIS, page 303.

- Reduce your risk of heart disease. See ATHEROSCLEROSIS, page 83.
- Adopt a program of regular exercise — at least 30 minutes five times a week.

In addition to your daily basic antioxidant vitamin/mineral supplement, take:

- Boron: 2 mg. daily.
- Calcium: 1200 mg. daily in the form of calcium citrate.
- Magnesium: 400 mg. daily.
- Vitamin E: 400 to 600 I.U. daily.
- Chromium: 100 mcg. three times a day.
- Dong quai, a Chinese herb available in health food stores. Take according to package directions.
- Black Cohosh: in the form of Remifemin the standard dosage is 2 tablets, twice daily.

CHAPTER 25

Migraine Headache

Migraines have been a scourge throughout recorded history, its victims including Socrates, Alexander the Great, and Napoleon. While the migraine sufferers noted by history are men, twice as many women as men suffer from migraine headaches. In fact, nearly 20 percent of all women are prone to migraines, with some suffering from daily attacks, while others have an attack every several months.

During a migraine attack, the blood vessels of the brain become swollen and cause irritation to the adjoining nerves. The debilitating effects of migraine are distinctly different from those of tension and sinus headaches which are caused, respectively, by tense muscles and swollen sinus tissues irritating the nerves. The typical migraine patient has suffered from more than one attack, and has a history of migraines in the family.

Symptoms Include:

- An unexplained feeling of depression or irritability, and an increased sensitivity to light and noise, which may precede the attack by several hours. These are caused by a preliminary constriction of the blood vessels of the brain.

- An "aura" of flashing lights or blind spots, and a feeling of being lightheaded just before the attack — a symptom experienced by many, but not all, migraine patients.

- An intense pain along one side of the head once the blood vessels of the head, constricted in the preliminary, or warning, stage, swell up. The one-sided aspect is specific to migraine, which comes from the Greek word for "half-a-skull."

- Intense nausea and vomiting frequently accompany migraines.

A predisposition to migraine is caused by an inherited instability of the vascular system — an instability which may also cause fainting spells and heighten the vasodilatory effects of various chemical agents. The blood platelets of migraine patients have been found to aggregate more readily in response to neurotransmitters such as serotonin and adrenaline than the blood platelets of the average individual. And the nervous system and the neurotransmitters it releases may also play a part.

A migraine attack is usually incapacitating. Medications to reduce pain are only marginally effective, and then only if taken before the attack.

Once the migraine starts, intense nausea sets in and the stomach shuts down. New prescription medications can stop an incipient attack, but still leave an aftermath of depletion and deep fatigue.

Fortunately, natural therapy is extremely effective in preventing migraines, once the cause of the migraines is known.

The Causes Of Migraines

Different things cause migraines in different people. What brings on your migraine may not affect another person predisposed to migraines, and the other way around. You may have to play detective to discover what triggers your migraines. I recommend that my patients keep a detailed diary for two or three weeks, or longer if the migraines are far apart — to record everything they eat, drink and do during that time.

I should note that it's as important to record the meals you skip as the ones you eat. Many of my patients have found this technique of keeping a diary very useful in determining what brings on their migraines and then eliminating the offending food, drink, or activity.

Sandra, an investment banker on Wall Street, used her laptop computer as her diary, keeping track of her day with the same zeal she used to keep track of her clients' investments. She had been plagued by migraines since her teens, and was electrified when I told her she could prevent the attacks once she identified the cause. Within two months she had pinpointed the trigger — low blood sugar in her case — and was able to prevent any further attacks by taking appropriate action.

Here are some frequent causes, or trigger points, for migraines.

1. **Sensitivity to Chemicals**: Chemicals in foods frequently trigger a migraine attack. Chemicals frequently implicated include:

- MSG, the flavor enhancer, and nitrates, used in bacon, hot dogs, and other preserved meats.
- Artificial sweeteners such as Aspartame, found in Nutrasweet.
- Amines, which are chemicals that dilate the blood vessels, and are naturally found in many foods.

Common Food Sources Of Amines	
Aged Meat	Eggplant
Avocado	Pineapple
Banana	Plum
Cabbage	Potato
Canned Fish	Tomato
Cheese	Wine And Beer
Cured Meat	Yeast Extract

2. **Sensitivity to Foods**: There are also foods which, while not containing amines, can trigger off a migraine if they provoke a reaction. Of course, if you detect a link between a food and the onset of a migraine, you must eliminate that food from your diet.

Allergenic Foods Implicated With Migraines

Apple	Fish	Rice
Beef	Goat's Milk	Rye
Benzoic Acid	Grapes	Soy
Caffeine	Oats	Tea
Cane Sugar	Onion	Tomato
Corn	Orange	Walnuts
Cow's Milk	Peanuts	Wheat
Egg	Pork	Yeast

---

3. **Low Blood Sugar** often triggers a migraine. A headache brought on by low blood sugar generally disappears once the sugar level is back up: i.e. following a meal. But for those prone to migraines, low blood sugar may trigger a reaction that sets off a full migraine attack. These can be prevented by regular meals eaten on a regular schedule, as well as chromium supplements, a chemical that helps to stabilize blood sugar. See also HYPOGLYCEMIA, page 243.

Janice, a patient whom I treated for hypoglycemia, was delighted to discover that her migraine headaches disappeared together with other problems caused by low blood sugar. The connection was reinforced one week when, having forgotten about her low blood sugar diet, she found the symptoms of hypoglycemia came back . . . followed by a migraine attack! Since that time, Janice, grown more cautious, has been free of migraines.

4. **Stress and Excitement** have been known to precipitate migraines. Exercise has been proved effective in avoiding stress induced migraines. A doctor at the Neurology Department of the New Mexico School of Medicine reported that several of his patients became free of migraines after jogging 7 to 9 miles a day, at a speed of seven to nine minutes per mile. I recommend that all of my patients with migraines adopt a daily exercise program. See STRESS CONTROL, page 321.

Luella, a patient of mine who had a difficult childhood and was still on tentative terms with her parents, realized that her migraine attacks were precipitated by any imminent family reunion. She discovered she could ward off the attack by swimming vigorously at the local Y the day before the dreaded visit. The exercise evidently served to block the release of the neurotransmitters provoked by anxiety and stress.

5. **Fluctuating Estrogen Levels** may explain why women suffer from migraines more frequently than men. Changing hormone levels in your menstrual cycle may be precipitating your migraines. Women who suffer pre-menstrual migraines are generally migraine free during their pregnancy, when hormone levels are constant. Birth control

hormone pills and estrogen replacement pills may also affect migraine activity.

If you suffer pre-menstrual migraines, it may be due to falling blood sugar levels. A hypoglycemia diet and chromium supplements are the preventive treatment. For menstrual muscle cramping that may bring on a headache, calcium and evening primrose oil will bring relief.

6. **Other Factors**, from changes in routine to environmental surroundings, can precipitate a migraine. If you get up late on weekends, have a change in working hours, or stay up late working on a project, you may precipitate a migraine. A change in climate can bring on a migraine, as can bright sunlight and bright artificial light, or staring too long at a computer or television screen. High winds and loud or high-pitched sounds have also been implicated with migraines.

Sometimes two different factors combine to fuse a migraine trigger. Stephanie, a graduate student plagued by frequent migraines, kept a diary for several weeks but was unable to determine a cause for her migraines until, reviewing her entries she discovered that there wasn't one cause. She could skip a meal most days without a problem. She could deal with fatigue and stress. But if she skipped a meal while she was under stress — for instance, prior to an exam, she would set off a migraine.

Watch That Diet Soda!

Some people are sensitive to artificial sweeteners like Aspartame, which is found in Nutrasweet. If you drink diet sodas regularly or use Nutrasweet regularly and you suffer from migraines, try eliminating all artificial sweeteners from your diet for a week or two to see if it eliminates your headaches.

Preventing Migraines

When you've identified the cause that triggers your migraine you can take appropriate corrective action. But whether or not you are able to determine a specific reason, there are additional things you can do to prevent a migraine.

Take Aspirin

Studies have found that one aspirin taken every other day cuts down the incidence of migraine headaches by reducing the aggregation of blood platelets. These platelets, when clumped together, produce serotonin, a neurotransmitter linked to migraines. Aggregated platelets also form the blood clots which lead to blood attacks, which is why aspirin, by "thinning" the blood, also cuts down the risk of heart attack.

Natural Supplements For Migraine

Feverfew, an herb that has long been used as a migraine treatment in Europe, has some of the same anti-inflammatory effects as aspirin without the side effects. A double-blind study of patients who had been helped by feverfew was conducted at the London Migraine Clinic. One test group, given a placebo instead of feverfew to determine if their migraine symptoms got worse, suffered worse migraine attacks, more often.

Fish oils, also known as omega-3's, have anti-inflammatory properties for a number of conditions, including migraines.

Magnesium deficiencies have been linked with migraines, and I recommend a magnesium supplement in the treatment of migraines.

> Sometimes people go for long periods thinking that they're suffering from migraine headaches when, in fact, they have chronic sinusitis which can cause regular, painful headaches. If you're uncertain whether you have a sinus problem or migraines, consult your doctor.

A Natural Treatment For Migraine Headaches

- Try to identify the cause of your migraine by keeping a daily food/activity diary. Especially note foods listed above as possible triggers of migraine headaches. You may be sensitive to a chemical in a food or you may have a food allergy that triggers your headaches. See if you can establish a pattern between something you ate or some unusual activity that caused your headache.

- Other migraine triggers include changes in routine, such as late rising on a holiday or change of working hours; changes in climate, high winds, loud or high-pitched sounds; bright sunlight or bright artificial light, and prolonged staring at television, movie or computer screens. Keep these triggers in mind when you compile your diary.

- Pay particular attention to the hormonal fluctuations of your menstrual cycle to see if your migraines are connected to changing estrogen levels. Headaches caused by low blood sugar can be helped by chromium. (See **PMS**, page 311 and HYPOGLYCEMIA, page 243.)

  - Chromium: 100 micrograms of the trivalent form three times daily.

- Headaches caused by muscle cramping can be helped by evening primrose oil and calcium. (See **PMS**, page 311.)
- Evening primrose oil: four 500 mg. capsules in morning and four 500 mg. capsules in evening. (Take evening primrose oil for five cycles and if no improvement, discontinue.)
- Calcium: 1200 mg. at bedtime.
- If you are post-menopausal and on estrogen replacement therapy, your medication could be a factor in your migraines. Discuss this with your doctor.
- Eat regular meals at regular times to avoid low blood sugar. Never skip meals. See HYPOGLYCEMIA, page 243.
- Keep stress under control with stress reducing techniques. See STRESS CONTROL, page 321.
- Adopt a regular exercise program.

In addition to your daily basic antioxidant vitamin/mineral supplement, take:

- One aspirin every other day.
- The herb feverfew: 150 mg. twice a day or as directed on package.
- Fish oils: 1000 mg. 3 times a day.
- Magnesium: 250 mg. twice daily.

CHAPTER 26

Mitral Valve Prolapse

Mitral valve prolapse is a common abnormality of the heart valve that controls the flow of blood between the left atrium and the left ventricle. In mitral valve prolapse, the valve billows back toward the ventricle each time the ventricle contracts, and there is a slight leaking of blood across the valve. On rare occasions, the leaking can be substantial and can even become life-threatening, but for the vast majority of patients mitral valve prolapse is a benign condition.

As a general rule, there are no symptoms associated with the condition, which a doctor usually discovers when he hears a slight heart murmur or click during a routine examination. But some people become so alarmed at the diagnosis that they start having panic attacks and palpitations, which of course alarms them all the more.

Deanna, a young artist who had recently been diagnosed with MVP, came to me complaining of anxiety, palpitations, headaches, breathlessness, weakness and chest pains. Since these are the symptoms that on occasion accompany the more serious form of the abnormality, I ordered an echocardiogram for Deanna. The results, when they came, clearly indicated that Deanna's MVP abnormality was so slight it would not produce any symptoms at all. The symptoms had been prompted by the deep anxiety most people feel when they believe they may have a heart problem.

When I told Deanna, she heaved a great sigh of relief. "I've been sick with worry," she said, "to the point I couldn't concentrate on anything else. So I have no cause for concern?"

I reassured Deanna that she didn't. A recent study found that 17 percent of the young women in the study had evidence of MVP, and that most of them, like Deanna, were women of slender build with long fingers, and a relatively shallow chest from front to back.

The condition is so common that some doctors feel it shouldn't be considered an abnormality, but merely a normal variant in heart structure. But it's interesting to note that women are more prone to it today than they were in previous generations: the same study found that among women over eighty years of age, only 1 percent had MVP.

The most common recommendation for people with MVP is to take antibiotics when undergoing surgery, or any medical procedure that may involve bleeding and cause infection in the heart valve. For instance, the prophylactic use of antibiotics is recommended for a routine cleaning at the dentist's, or for an infected cut or wound.

I explained these precautions to Deanna, and recommended that she get periodic checkups. In the course of an average lifetime, as the heart undergoes more than three billion contractions, the valve is subject to deterioration. To prevent damage to the heart, I recommended Coenzyme Q-10 and magnesium supplements to Deanna and, since her symptoms had been brought on by anxiety, I suggested that she should use stress control techniques.

Low Blood Sugar And MVP

I should mention, low blood sugar will sometimes cause symptoms that patients believe is caused by their MVP. If you have MVP, and suffer from occasional headaches, weakness and anxiety, try to determine if your symptoms are brought on by low blood sugar, or hypoglycemia. See HYPOGLYCEMIA, page 243. A word of warning: MVP is usually symptomless, and only a doctor can diagnose a mitral valve prolapse condition. If you believe you have MVP, ask your doctor to do an echocardiogram.

If you do have MVP, I recommend that you use the natural therapy approach outlined below to protect your heart and gain control over stress and anxiety.

Keep Stress Under Control

It's important to keep in mind that MVP is a very common condition with few risks or side effects. To keep panic attacks at bay, I recommend that people with MVP should:

- Adopt a regular exercise program to promote fitness and help you relax.
- Use stress control techniques such as progressive relaxation. See STRESS CONTROL, page 321.

Use Natural Supplements

Coenzyme Q-10 is very helpful to people with heart conditions, including MVP, because it strengthens the heart and promotes exercise tolerance. One interesting study showed that 50–75 percent of people with heart disease had abnormally low levels of Co Q-10.

Magnesium helps to regulate the heartbeat, and control palpitations. It's an important supplement for people with MVP.

A Natural Treatment For Mitral Valve Prolapse

- Your MVP will have been identified by a doctor who will inform you as to the severity (or lack of it) of your condition and will recommend appropriate treatment if necessary.

In addition to your daily basic antioxidant vitamin/mineral supplement, take:

- Coenzyme Q-10: 30 mg. three times daily.
- Magnesium: 400 mg. daily.

Also:

- Be sure that any symptoms you have are not a result of low blood sugar. (See HYPOGLYCEMIA, page 243.)
- Make sure that you have a regular exercise program to reduce stress and that you are familiar with stress reducing techniques. (See STRESS CONTROL, page 321.)

CHAPTER 27

Morning Sickness

Several of my pregnant patients have complained about having morning sickness. Lucille, for instance, who had come to see me about her carpal tunnel syndrome, mentioned that she was two months pregnant and suffering from "morning sickness" that lasted all day long. Her gynecologist had told her the nausea would disappear by the end of the first trimester, but she had another month to go and it felt like an eternity.

I was glad to tell Lucille there are several natural therapies that are very effective against nausea and vomiting.

The first thing, of course, is to avoid heavy, greasy foods which are difficult to digest. Eat frequently to keep your stomach full, and have some protein with each meal or snack, because protein takes longer to digest than carbohydrates. Since an empty stomach in the morning will aggravate your nausea, keep some crackers at your bedside for a morning snack before you get up.

If you have severe nausea or vomiting, and cannot keep your food down for three days, you must see your doctor. But the following techniques will help you to relieve regular nausea and morning sickness.

Some women are nauseated as a result of their pre-natal vitamins. (Many people are nauseated by any vitamin that they take on an empty stomach or first thing in the morning.) Try taking your vitamin after breakfast, right after dinner or right before bedtime if this is your problem.

Try Acupressure

Some people swear by acupressure as a means of preventing nausea. There are acupressure points located on the inside of the wrist, about three finger-widths toward the elbow. If you apply pressure to these points, which are called "neiguan," you can relieve feelings of nausea. You can use your thumb and fingers, or buy "seasickness straps" at a marine store, pharmacy, or health food store. These straps have little bumps that press on the correct points and can be worn at any time.

Natural Supplements For Morning Sickness

Many of my patients have found relief from nausea by taking B^6 supplements, and several studies have shown the supplements are very effective in relieving nausea and vomiting in the early stages of pregnancy.

> **IMPORTANT**
> Since B^6 supplementation can affect nursing, do not take B^6 supplements after the first three months of pregnancy.

Ginger is another supplement that can be very helpful in easing the symptoms of morning sickness. Ginger is a time-honored remedy for upset stomachs, including nausea and seasickness. I particularly recommend it to pregnant women because it does not have any of the side effects that drug treatment can have. Ginger capsules are available at health food stores.

A Natural Treatment For Nausea In Pregnancy

- Take 50 mg. of Vitamin B^6 daily for seven days. If no relief, discontinue. In any event, discontinue after the first six weeks of pregnancy as B^6 can cause difficulty in nursing.
- Take ginger capsules: 250 mg. three times daily.
- Apply pressure to the acupressure points on the wrist. Measure three fingerwidths

up the inside of the wrist from the crease and press for several minutes, or invest in a "seasickness band" from a marine supply store.

- Avoid greasy foods.
- Have frequent protein snacks.
- Keep your stomach full.

CHAPTER 28

Osteoporosis

Osteoporosis, which means "porous bones" in Latin, is a crippling condition that affects millions of elderly people. Osteoporosis sets in when the diet is deficient in calcium, and the body draws on the bones for the calcium it needs for various metabolic processes. When calcium is leached from the bones, they lose strength and resiliency, eventually becoming brittle and thin.

Women with advanced osteoporosis lose inches in height, bowed under the body weight that their spines grow too weak to support. They are at risk of bone fractures that can leave them hospitalized, sometimes for life.

Each year, half a million people, most of them women, are hospitalized after breaking a hip weakened by osteoporosis. One quarter of them will never go home again, but will remain hospitalized or be placed in a nursing home. Bones weakened by osteoporosis become so frail that it is not uncommon for someone to fracture a rib simply by coughing. The bright side of this grim picture is that you can prevent osteoporosis — and even reverse its effects — by consuming an adequate amount of calcium and other nutrients, and by adopting a program of regular exercise.

Women are at higher risk of osteoporosis than men because they have less bone mass to begin with, and because they lose it faster after menopause. If you are a woman of fifty-five, or if you are in one of the high-risk categories, you should follow my natural therapy guidelines to prevent osteoporosis.

Women At Highest Risk For Osteoporosis

- Asian women
- White women, especially blond or redheaded women of Northern European ancestry
- Postmenopausal women
- Underweight women
- Women with small bone structure
- Heavy alcohol users
- Smokers
- Women on a high protein diet
- Women with a family history of osteoporosis
- Women who experienced menopause before the age of forty
- Women who are diabetic
- Women with thyroid disease
- Women with asthma or other lung disease
- Women who take glucocorticoids (for example, cortisone or prednisone prescribed for rheumatoid arthritis)

Monitor Your Calcium Intake

I believe that every woman, whether or not she is in a high risk category, should make sure she gets enough calcium throughout her life. Starting in her teens, she should consume at least 1200 mg. of calcium daily: that's roughly the equivalent of four glasses of milk. If she's nursing, or when she reaches menopause, this amount should be increased to 1500 mg. (The additional calcium is needed to compensate for the decrease in estrogen, the female hormone necessary to deliver calcium to the bone.)

Since it's unlikely that most women can drink sufficient milk to supply them with the needed calcium amount, I recommend that all my women patients take calcium supplements in the recommended amounts.

Which Calcium Supplement?

When you're looking for a calcium supplement, you may well be confused by the large variety of calciums to choose from. There is calcium lactate, and calcium phosphate, and calcium gluconate, and calcium carbonate. I don't recommend any of them, as the body has trouble absorbing them.

Instead, I recommend you choose calcium citrate, which is very well absorbed and is not expensive. The best time to take your calcium supplement is at bedtime, because research shows that's when it's best absorbed. As a bonus, calcium at bedtime will help you to get a good night's sleep!

I believe that women should also increase their calcium consumption through their diet. Skim milk, nonfat yogurt, green vegetables, and sardines with bones are all excellent sources of calcium.

SOURCES OF CALCIUM	
Food	**mg. Of Calcium**
Yogurt, plain, nonfat, 8 oz.	452
Yogurt, plain, low fat, 8 oz.	414
Nonfat dry milk, 1/4 cup dry	377
Collard greens, frozen, cooked, 1 cup	357
Sardines, with bones, 3 1/4	351
1 percent milk, protein fortified, 8 oz.	349
Whole milk, 8 oz.	291
Spinach, frozen, cooked, 1 cup	278
Cheese, goat, hard, 1 oz.	254
Calcium-enriched orange juice, 8 oz.	225
Cheese, cheddar, 1 oz.	204
Cheese, muenster, 1 oz.	203
Salmon, canned, with bones, 3 oz.	203
Cheese, mozzarella, part skim, 1 oz.	183
Kale, frozen, cooked, 1 cup	179
Broccoli, cooked, chopped, 1 cup	178
Mustard greens, cooked, chopped, 1 cup	150
Cheese, feta, 1 oz.	140
Oysters, 1 cup	111
Chard, cooked, chopped, 1 cup	102
Cheese, goat, semi-soft, 1 oz.	84
Cheese, cottage, creamed, 4 oz.	68
Source: U.S. Department of Agriculture	

Nutritional Supplements For Osteoporosis

There are other minerals and vitamins you must supplement in addition to calcium:

Magnesium, a mineral involved in calcium metabolism, is critical in fighting osteoporosis. In one study, women who received half the recommended amount of calcium, and double the recommended dose of magnesium, gained bone density at a rate *sixteen* times greater than women who received counseling, but no supplements.

Vitamin D is also important to supplement. Deficiencies of Vitamin D can promote bone loss. If you're taking a good vitamin supplement which contains 400 I.U. of vitamin D, you don't need to take more.

Boron is a mineral that reduces the excretion of calcium from the body. It's wise to take a boron supplement to reduce chances of developing osteoporosis.

There are other supplements that have a positive effect on calcium retention but they are needed in such minute quantities that I tell my patients to simply rely on a good daily multiple vitamin/mineral supplement.

If Your Problem With Osteoporosis Is Severe. . .

There's a drug called Etidronate, approved by the FDA for a different bone disorder, that has proved helpful in fighting osteoporosis when taken with calcium. Discuss this drug with your doctor.

It's Not Only About Calcium. . .

Reduced calcium consumption isn't the only factor that affects bone loss. Certain foods actually cause the body to lose calcium. They act like calcium bandits that rob your bones of this critical mineral. A diet high in protein foods increases calcium excretion and therefore bone loss. Many people today are restricting their protein intake by eating less meat and I recommend this trend.

Of course meat isn't the only protein: fish and chicken are also protein foods. The point is to reduce your overall protein intake. Six ounces per day — the equivalent of a small chicken breast or a small fish fillet — is really enough.

Caffeine can also cause calcium loss from the body. If you drink more than one cup of coffee or tea per day, you're ingesting a chemical that's actually acting to leach calcium from your bones. I tell my patients to limit coffee consumption to no more than one caffeinated drink per day. And be sure that any carbonated drinks you consume don't have caffeine as an ingredient.

Alcohol can also leach calcium from your body so limit your consumption. I believe that, to maintain optimum health, it's best to avoid alcohol entirely but certainly no more than two to three drinks per week.

Did you need to know another bad thing about cigarettes? Well, they lower estrogen levels in women, thereby increasing a woman's risk of developing osteoporosis. Moreover, smokers have been found to have double the risk of back fractures of non-smokers.

Exercise Is Essential

Exercise is essential to maintaining, and even restoring, bone density. Exercise, in conjunction with sufficient dietary calcium, virtually eliminates the risk of osteoporosis. It does not need to be strenuous exercise, but it needs to be regular. A daily walk of half an hour a day will do the trick. Also, lifting has been found to increase bone density, so when you're carrying your suitcases or groceries you have the satisfaction of knowing you're warding off osteoporosis.

How to Have Healthy Bones for Life

Birth to Age 35: Build your bones to their peak density and strength by means of a a calcium-rich diet plus weight bearing exercise.

Age 35 to 50 (or menopause): Your goal during this period is to maintain the bone mass you've got. You should take at least 1000 mg. of calcium a day, do weight bearing exercise, limit alcohol to one or two drinks daily, stop smoking, avoid any drastic diets and limit or eliminate caffeine.

Age 50 (or menopause) and over: During the first few years after menopause, your bone density plummets and, to compound the problem, your calcium absorption becomes less efficient. Take at least 1500 mg. of calcium daily, continue to exercise, continue optimum lifestyle and consider hormone replacement therapy if indicated.

A Natural Treatment For Osteoporosis

- Increase foods containing calcium, including nonfat or low fat dairy products. You can add dry, powdered milk to certain recipes — puddings, meatloaves, muffins and baked goods — to boost calcium content.

- Reduce or eliminate the following from your diet:
  - Too much protein — limit yourself to 6 ounces per day
  - Caffeine
  - Smoking
  - Excess alcohol
  - Salt (avoid the salt shaker; use only in cooking)
  - Sugar

In addition to your daily basic antioxidant vitamin/mineral, take:

- Calcium: 1200 mg. of calcium citrate at bedtime.
- Magnesium: 400 mg. daily.
- Boron: 3 mg. daily.
- A good multiple vitamin which will provide 400 I.U. of Vitamin D.

Also

- Adopt a program of regular exercise.

CHAPTER 29

PMS

Brett, a new patient who was telling me about her recent health history, had a long list of symptoms and complaints. She often felt irritable and tense. She had a tendency to bloating — "puffing up like a blowfish," is the way she put it. Her breasts would get so tender she had trouble sleeping. She often had headaches. She often had food cravings, particularly for sweets. At this point, Brett stopped and grinned at me. She was a highly attractive and energetic young woman in her last year of college, who at that moment seemed in the best of health.

"You must think I'm a hypochondriac," said Brett.

What I thought — and later confirmed — was that Brett was suffering from premenstrual syndrome.

PMS was first recognized in medical literature in 1931, but its wide diversity of symptoms, which can vary greatly from one woman to another, can make it difficult to diagnose. There may be as many as 150 symptoms that women can suffer one or two weeks before their menstrual period, which means of course that some women don't feel their best for almost half the month. The severity of the symptoms also vary from one woman to another, from mildly annoying to extreme. In one well-publicized case PMS was used as a defense to murder.

Recent research indicates that hormonal imbalances, prostaglandin imbalance and vitamin and mineral imbalances are the causes of PMS. I believe that the most effective way to treat PMS is to address these imbalances and correct them through natural therapy, rather than prescribe drugs that may merely mask some of the symptoms. In fact, the drug most frequently prescribed for PMS, progesterone, has recently been found ineffective in its treatment.

Brett told me that, midway through her menstrual cycle, she would start experiencing symptoms which would grow more severe as the period approached. None of them were incapacitating, but they were annoying. She particularly deplored the mood swings which made it difficult for her to concentrate on her work, and was delighted to hear about the amino acid DL-phenylalanine, a supplement that has been near miraculous in combating the PMS moodiness of some of my patients.

I also recommended that Brett use a combined approach of diet, exercise and additional supplements to combat PMS, not just to treat the symptoms, but to address the underlying biochemical imbalances that had caused them in the first place.

Two months later, when Brett came back to see me, I was glad to hear that the PMS natural therapy had worked for her as well.

"The mood swings pretty much disappeared, just as you predicted," Brett told me. "But what I really found amazing is that, for the first time in years, I didn't crave sweets in the middle of the month. It's heaven not to have to agonize about whether or not to make a trip to the candy bar machine."

Diet And PMS

Diet plays an important part in treating PMS because it helps to regulate blood sugar levels, which fluctuate in PMS patients. As with most of my other patients who suffer from PMS, Brett hadn't realized that her mid-month sugar cravings were a natural response to physiological changes in her body.

After ovulation, which generally occurs mid-month in the cycle, a change in the insulin-binding capacity of the cells brings on a related change in the body's response to sugar in the diet. Once you control blood sugar levels with diet and chromium supplements, most of the symptoms of PMS naturally disappear.

If you suffer from any of the symptoms of PMS, the natural therapy treatment will help you eliminate them, and replace them with increased energy and well-being.

Blood Sugar And PMS

Many of my patients have been surprised to find that, once they give up sugar in their diet, their sugar cravings disappear. Giving up sugar doesn't just mean giving up the sugar bowl: it means eliminating candy, cookies, cakes, frosted cereals and so on.

One you stop ingesting refined sugar, you will reduce the production of insulin and stop the sugar/insulin yo-yo effect which places heavy demands on your body.

Regular meals at regular times will also help you regulate blood sugar. Be sure to have enough protein with each meal to provide adequate energy until the next one.

In addition, I recommend chromium supplements to my patients. Chromium is very helpful in stabilizing blood sugar levels, and many people have marginal deficiencies, particularly if they are athletic, or drink a lot of coffee or tea. A large amount of sugar intake also depletes chromium from the body. For more information, refer to HY-POGLYCEMIA, page 243.

Improve Your Nutritional Status

Research has shown that dietary fat is linked with prostaglandin and plasma estrogen levels. You can influence PMS symptoms by the type and amount of fat your use in your diet. Animal fats worsen the symptoms of PMS, and the more animal fat you eat, the worse you will feel. The "good" fats, on the other hand, which are olive oil, safflower and canola oil, tend to reduce the symptoms of PMS.

Salt also has a role in PMS by causing the retention of fluid which is, of course, responsible for a bloated feeling and breast tenderness. Further, salt can create a stronger insulin reaction to sugar, thus promoting the low blood sugar levels which cause weakness and irritability.

Fiber, on the other hand, plays a beneficial role in PMS by helping to clear excessive estrogen, which aggravates the symptoms, from the intestinal system. Increase your intake of fiber for at least two weeks prior to your menstrual period.

Caffeine plays an adversarial role in PMS. To begin with, caffeine affects the same adenosine receptors in the brain which also receive progesterone and other hormones, and heightens their effect. Also, caffeine contributes to changes in blood sugar levels, and stimulates production of stress hormones, all of which heighten the symptoms of PMS.

Studies have linked the amount of caffeine ingested to the severity of PMS symptoms. Women in Boston, as well as women in China, who drank coffee and caffeinated drinks were found to have more aggravated PMS symptoms than women who didn't.

For additional information on nutrition, please refer to A HEALTHY WOMAN'S DAILY ROUTINE, page 19.

Try Nutritional Supplements For PMS

A USDA study conducted in 1985 found that the majority of women are below the RDA recommended levels in vitamins and minerals. Of these, 87 percent were deficient in Vitamin E, 74 percent were deficient in calcium, 56 percent in iron, and 46 percent in folacin. That may explain why so many women suffer from PMS, and why their symptoms are relieved with vitamin supplements. I recommend:

- **The B complex** for stabilizing hormone levels and fighting stress. Also B^6 to help relieve fluid retention.

- **Vitamin A** — in doses no higher than recommended in Natural Treatment For PMS at the end of this chapter. High doses of Vitamin A are unsafe when used over a long period of time and without medical supervision.

- **Vitamin E**, which promotes some of the prostaglandins that inhibit prolactin, known to aggravate PMS. Vitamin E greatly improves breast swelling and tenderness, and is even helpful in fibrocystic disease.

- **Calcium and magnesium**, which reduce depression, irritability, headaches, mood swings, cramps and back pain.

- **Zinc**, which relieves all PMS symptoms, and premenstrual acne in particular. An interesting study showed that women without PMS take twice the amount of zinc as women with the syndrome.

- **Evening primrose oil** relieves cramping, irritability, breast discomfort, anxiety, tiredness, as well as swollen fingers and ankles. Evening primrose oil is somewhat slow to take effect: while it's somewhat helpful starting with the first cycle, its full effects will be felt with the fifth cycle on the supplement.

- **Vitamin C**, which helps to regulate the clearance of estrogen from the body.

- **DL-phenylalanine**, the amino acid I mentioned earlier. It's used in the production of certain neurotransmitters and has been extremely helpful in fighting mood swings, and severe depression and moodiness in particular.

Exercise Is Helpful

It's long been known that women who work out regularly, including professional dancers and professional athletes, suffer infrequently from PMS. A recent study showed that women who exercise moderately for a full cycle experience less premenstrual fluid retention, breast tenderness, and depression.

Exercise promotes the production of endorphin, which alleviates or eliminates PMS symptoms. One of my PMS patients who started walking for about half an hour each day reported that she had her first menstrual period not preceded by PMS.

A Natural Treatment For PMS

Diet

- Follow a low fat diet.
- Eliminate sweets.
- Eat regular meals at regular times.
- Eat protein at lunch and dinner (fish, chicken, tuna, turkey).
- Limit alcohol.
- Limit salt.
- Limit dairy products.
- Limit caffeine to no more than one caffeinated drink per day.
- Increase complex carbohydrates, including green leafy vegetables, legumes, whole grains and cereals, to increase fiber.
- Increase intake of olive or safflower oil.

In addition to your daily basic antioxidant vitamin/mineral supplement, take all of these supplements for three months and if there is no improvement in symptoms, discontinue:

- Vitamin A: 10,000 to 25,000 I.U. daily.
- Vitamin B^6: 100 mg. three times a day for two weeks prior to period.
- Vitamin C: 1000 mg. daily.

- Vitamin E: 400 — 800 I.U. daily.
- Magnesium: 400 mg. daily.
- Chromium: 100 micrograms of trivalent chromium three times a day.
- Zinc: 50 mg. daily.
- Evening primrose oil: four 500 mg. capsules in morning and four 500 mg. capsules in evening. (Take evening primrose oil for five cycles and if no improvement, discontinue).
- DL-phenylalanine: one or two 500 mg. capsules three times a day.

Lifestyle

- Adopt a regular exercise program.

CHAPTER 30 ——— *Stress Control*

We're just beginning to understand the full impact of mental and emotional stress upon the human body. Stress and its effects are not imaginary — they are as quantifiable as the emissions of a faulty automobile engine, and potentially as deadly.

Stress causes the release of a number of powerful biochemicals into the system. Over a period of time, these biochemicals will weaken and break down the weakest links in the system. Thus, some people start to suffer from multiple allergies and colds. Others develop serious problems of the digestive system. People with headaches will find they'll be greatly aggravated. And disease of the circulatory system can be dangerously aggravated by stress.

Indeed, population studies have demonstrated that increased stress brought on by death, divorce

— or even a job change — is linked to an increased risk of death from heart disease.

That's why I was concerned about Emily. I had not seen her for ten years or so, when, while still in law school, she came to my office about an annoying allergic rash. Now she was in her early thirties, divorced, with two small children, and a job in the District Attorney's office.

She told me she'd been suffering from headaches that were interfering with her job. She had trouble sleeping at night, and her allergic rashes had returned. But what Emily hadn't realized was that her blood pressure was sharply higher than it should be at her age. She seemed tense and angry, pacing up and down my office as though it were a cage.

"Angry?" she said in answer to my question. "Maybe I am. Why wouldn't I be? My ex hasn't come up with child support for six months, my department is so understaffed we each have to do the work of three people, and my children are closer to the babysitter than they are to me. And the plumber still hasn't showed up to fix the leaky toilet."

After I completed my examination, Emily was taken aback to hear that her blood pressure had escalated to potentially dangerous levels. Further, since her cholesterol count was well within the normal range, there was good reason to believe that her hypertension was brought on by stress, which might also be causing her other symptoms. I reminded Emily that the rash she had suffered while in law school had disappeared spontaneously, shortly after she had passed her bar examinations.

Fight Or Flight

"You mean my problems are psychosomatic?" Emily wanted to know. She seemed to think that the effects of stress were abstract, confined to the realms of the mind and imagination. Like many of my patients who suffer from stress, Emily didn't understand that the body is programmed to respond to stress with a complex series of biochemical changes intended to mobilize an instantaneous reaction, known as the "fight-or-flight" response.

The adrenal glands release various hormones including epinephrine and norepinephrine to energize the body. The heartbeat quickens, the reflexes are sharpened, the nervous system's sensitivity becomes acute. The muscles tense, the pupils dilate, and the blood vessels contract so as to retain heat and force more blood into the major organs. The liver releases stored glucose to provide energy for the fight. The digestive system shuts down to conserve energy. To prevent blood loss in the battle, blood coagulation is heightened.

All of these mechanisms made more sense fifty thousand years ago, when we were running for our life toward our home cave, than they do today, while fuming over a billing error by a credit card company. Our automatic response to stress is really a primitive response, inappropriate to the modern world. *The purpose and goal of stress control is to change — not the outside stress stimuli, but our response to them.*

Emily couldn't understand why the effects of stress didn't disappear when the stressful agent was removed. Why would she develop a headache over an office problem that took place two days ago, she wanted to know. Of course, Emily was assuming that the biochemicals triggered at the time of stress were quickly disbursed the moment the stimulus was over. But that isn't so. An interesting experiment showed that mice who felt stressed by a flight from Boston to Seattle took three days to eliminate dangerous levels of adrenaline, cortisol, and other chemicals from their body.

In the case of the human body, we recover quickly from a one-time, stressful stimulus, such as a near accident in heavy traffic. But when the stress becomes a constant, as it often does over a job, an unhappy relationship, or a pile of unpaid bills, then your body has no opportunity to revert to normal. Instead, it goes into what Hans Selye, known as the father of stress theory, calls the "stage of resistance," in which the body tries to adapt to the constant stress.

Eventually, if the burden is not lightened, the body enters the "exhaustion stage." Here is where things begin to break down, and the body exhibits minor symptoms of disease. Some doctors believe that many ailments, including cancer and diseases of the immune system, are promoted by stress.

I told Emily she was an ideal candidate for stress control techniques. I believed that, if she got her stress under control, her blood pressure would decrease to normal levels and her overall health would improve. Emily, somewhat dubiously, agreed to try out my recommendations.

One month later, Emily reported she was sleeping better, and her rash had gone. I was pleased but not surprised that her blood pressure had gone down significantly. "I thought a lot about it," she told me, "and realized I had been allowing things to get to me. And it's not fair to my boys."

She had been practicing her relaxation response and it seemed to be working for her. She had also tried aromatherapy — "I don't know if it works, but it's fun," — and unwinding to music after the children were in bed. Emily still had the same problems and frustrations to deal with — she still had the same frustrations on her job, and her husband still hadn't made child support payments — but she was learning to control her response.

"I realize I still have a long way to go, but at least I'm beginning to control my stress, instead of having it control me," she said.

As several of my patients have remarked, once you admit that you're caught up in a spiral of stress you can learn to control it. You cannot eliminate all stress from your life. In all my years of medical practice I have never met anyone who was totally free of outside stress. I don't think such a condition is possible or even desirable. But it is possible to change our reactions to stress. Instead of the "fight-or-flight" response that was once useful to our cavemen ancestors, we can adopt one that's more suitable to our current times.

The Relaxation Response

After researching different methods of relaxation for myself and my patients, I selected the "relaxation response" method developed by Dr. Herbert Benson, a cardiologist associated with the Harvard Medical School and chief of the Section on Behavioral Medicine at New England Deaconess Hospital. Dr. Benson was one of the pioneers in the field of meditation, reporting on the connection between meditation and reduced blood pressure, as well as the reduced use of anti-hypertension drugs.

He used his knowledge of yoga, Sufism, Zen, Judaism, and Christianity to develop "relaxation response," a technique that can be used to achieve a quiet mind and a peaceful heart. Some of my patients thought the technique was too simple to be effective but after trying it, they were amazed that such a simple exercise could have such a calming and invigorating effect on their mind and body.

Relaxation response countermands the "fight-or-flight" response by producing directly opposite physiological reactions. It decreases your metabolism, your heart rate, your breathing rate and the activity of your sympathetic nervous system. It increases the alpha brain waves associated with feelings of relaxation and well-being, and decreases the blood flow to your muscles, as well as your blood lactate levels which are associated with fatigue. These changes are very different from the changes experienced by the body when you are sitting, or asleep.

I believe relaxation response works best when done twice a day, once in the middle of the day and once in the evening. Many of my patients do it just before or after lunch at their desks or at home, and again just after work.

To Invoke The Relaxation Response, You Will Need:

1. A quiet environment without noises or distractions. This can be anywhere: home, office, or hotel room. Many of my patients sit at their desk and invoke the R.R. One man told me that his gym has a "nap room" where people can rest and he uses that.

2. A mental device. The equivalent of using a mantra for meditation, this is a single-syllable word, or sound, that you repeat while meditating. It helps you to remove yourself from logical thought and distractions. Dr. Benson suggests the word "one." I have a patient who uses "snow" in the summer and "sun" in the winter.

3. A passive attitude. This just means not focusing on how well you're doing in the exercise or whether you are getting the correct response. When either of these thoughts occurs to you, let it go and focus instead on repeating your chosen word.

4. A comfortable position. You want to reduce awareness of your muscles as much as possible. A comfortable chair that supports your head is good. It's even better if you lie down.

The Relaxation Response Techniques

Once you have selected your "quiet environment" and are sitting or lying down in a comfortable position, you are ready to start the R.R. technique:

- Close your eyes.
- Relax your muscles. Start with the muscles in your feet, then your calves, thighs, lower torso, chest, shoulders, arms, neck, and head. Pay special attention to the muscles in your neck and face, which get very tense.
- Breathe through your nose, paying attention to your breathing. As you exhale, say aloud or just think about your chosen word.
- Do this for at least ten minutes — twenty, if you can. You can open your eyes to check the time, but Dr. Benson cautions against setting an alarm clock.

Try Aromatherapy

Some of my patients swear that aromatherapy is helpful for stress control, and indeed people have known since ancient times that scent can have a powerful effect on mood and emotion. Aromatherapy is prevalent in Japan, and is becoming popular in this country.

A recent study found that lavender was as effective as sleeping pills in helping elderly individuals get a good night's sleep. Sage and juniper berry oils are believed to relieve tension and lift one's spirits, while a relaxing blend of two drops of geranium, lavender, and sandalwood oils and one drop of ylang ylang oil can be used in a bath, massage, or a vaporizer for stress reduction. Rosemary oil, on the other hand, is used to stimulate the mind and body when a person is overworked.

Music Therapy for Stress Control

Some of my patients believe that music helps to unwind, and indeed the powerful emotional and stress reduction properties of music have been long appreciated. In modern times, researchers have discovered that certain natural rhythms and sounds, such as birds chirping, soft breezes or gurgling streams, produce soothing effects.

According to the American Institute of Stress, music has been widely used to alleviate stress and anxiety, to promote care and healing of coronary patients, and as an aid in treating headaches, digestive complaints, and various other disorders aggravated by emotional tension and stress.

CHAPTER 31

Tension Headaches

Most people know exactly what a tension headache feels like and if they didn't they'd quickly figure it out from all the commercials that feature people in the grip of one. The pain of a tension headache is felt in the forehead, temples, or the entire head. Your head feels tight, your neck rigid — the muscles in your neck and face are knotted and tense. This tension itself is the cause of your headache, because your tense muscles are irritating the sensitive nerve endings.

A migraine headache, on the other hand, is caused by swollen blood vessels pressing against the nerve endings, and a sinus headache is brought on by inflamed and swollen sinus tissue.

Many of my patients suffer with a tension headache from time to time, which is not surprising given the amount of sensory overload we have to deal with: heavy traffic, loud noise, blinding lights, harsh, unpleasant smells. But if you have repeated headaches occurring on particular days or at a particular place, you may be able to pinpoint the specific cause.

Many headaches are job-related, of course. When you work against a deadline and your work requires a high degree of accuracy, you are at increased risk of tension headaches because of the multiple stress factors.

Air traffic controllers, for instance, are said to suffer from frequent tension headaches. Heart surgeons, on the other hand, are not particularly given to headaches, perhaps because, while their work demands high accuracy and skill, they are not under pressure to get the job done within a specific time.

One of my long-time patients, Gianna, started having almost daily headaches when an organizational change placed a new boss at the head of her advertising department. Promoted beyond his level of ability, he turned out to be a rather stupid, unpleasant human being whose idea of management was to rant and scream at his employees, at the same time that he took credit for their work. Gianna decided not to quit — "he won't be there long at this rate," she predicted, but the daily tension headaches were making it difficult for her to do her work and deal with her clients.

I recommended that Gianna try the relaxation techniques described in this chapter to diffuse the tension which brought on her headaches. Gianna found the neck rolls, which only took a minute or two, were particularly helpful in relaxing her muscles. A brisk walk at lunchtime was also helpful. In addition Gianna signed up at a gym and started working out at lunchtime on any day she wasn't taking a client out to lunch.

Later, when she got home, she would take a warm bath before spending fifteen minutes or so on "progressive relaxation." Gianna told me these simple techniques effectively ended her headaches, and she liked them so well that she continued doing them long after the new boss was demoted to a different area.

There are other causes for tension headaches besides stress. A weak neck and back can bring on tension headaches, which can be relieved through exercises to strengthen the supporting muscles. A bad bite that causes tension in the jaw — known as temporomandibular pressure — can also cause headaches, and may require the attention of an orthodontist.

Caffeine Headaches

Coffee withdrawal can also cause tension headaches after you give up caffeine. Margaret, one of my patients who drank several cups of coffee on weekday mornings, suffered what I call "weekend" headaches because she tended to sleep in on weekends and didn't have her first cup of coffee until noon. The headaches she suffered on Saturday and Sunday afternoon were due to caffeine withdrawal.

I told Margaret to try cutting down her weekday coffee intake to one cup, so as to gradually wean herself from her caffeine addiction. She did, and also started getting up and having her cup of coffee earlier on weekends, and her headaches totally cleared up!

Headache Rebound

It's unfortunate that the painkillers people take for headaches can actually be the cause of more headaches. Many painkillers contain caffeine, and become the source of caffeine dependence and withdrawal. When you take them you feel better, but only because you fed your caffeine habit.

Steady users of aspirin or acetaminophen can also become overly dependent on the medication, and develop an "analgesic rebound headache" when it's withdrawn.

I recommend you limit your use of over-the-counter pain medication to no more than three times a week, and no more than four tablets a day.

> I've noticed that a few patients who complain of regular tension headaches and also chew gum routinely found that, when I suggested they stop chewing gum, their headaches disappeared. The constant tightening of the jaw muscles can bring on headaches.

Headaches And Low Blood Sugar

And then there are patients whose afternoon headaches were caused by low blood sugar. Their headaches cleared up when they gave up sugar and started eating regular meals which included protein. For more information about HYPOGLYCEMIA, please turn to page 243.

Food Sensitivities And Headaches

Food sensitivities that can cause migraine headaches can also cause tension headaches. The difference is that, with tension headaches, it's the muscles, and not the blood vessels, that are affected. For more information on allergenic foods, please refer to MIGRAINES, page 281.

> Most people have heard of "Chinese Restaurant Syndrome," where you get a headache shortly after eating at a Chinese restaurant. The headache is caused by a sensitivity to monosodium glutamate (MSG), a common ingredient in Chinese foods. The cure is simple: avoid foods containing MSG.

Relaxation Techniques For Headaches

To clear up your headaches you must, of course, address the problem that caused them in the first place. But whatever the reason, you can feel better and help prevent a recurrence by using the relaxation techniques outlined below.

- Stretch your muscles every hour or so during the day. Stretch, breathe deeply, and do a few neck rolls: you will feel your tense neck and upper shoulder muscles stretching as you do! You can also massage the back of your neck, pressing deeply into the tightly knotted muscles.

- Do "progressive relaxation," a yoga-like technique which consists of relaxing groups of muscles at one time, starting at the feet, and moving upward until you reach the head. For more information on progressive relaxation, please turn to STRESS CONTROL, page 321.

- Use heat on those tense muscles. A soak in a hot bath will do wonders, as will a long hot shower. Or you can use a heating pad.

- Take a nap if you can, or just lie quietly, eyes closed.

- Take a brisk walk to increase your circulation and oxygen flow.

Exercise And Headaches

Regular exercise diffuses tension and is one of the most effective ways of preventing tension headaches. Set up a program of exercise tailored to your level of fitness. In addition, incorporate daily stretching exercises into your exercise schedule.

A Natural Treatment For Tension Headaches

- Learn what triggers your headaches, including such things as sensory overload: shrill, persistent noise, harsh lights, feelings of claustrophobia, working against a deadline or performing a job where accuracy is essential.

- When you face any of these triggers be sure to use relaxation techniques to fight tension. Stretch muscles periodically, once every half-hour, and massage the neck and shoulders. See STRESS CONTROL, page 321.

- See MIGRAINE HEADACHE (page 281) to learn if your headaches are connected to food allergies or sensitivities.

- Use moist heat to relieve pain: take a warm shower or bath or use a moist (or dry) heating pad on your neck.

- Take a nap.

- Take a brisk walk.

- Adopt a program of regular exercise.

- Investigate whether jaw clenching or improper alignment of the jaw could be causing your headaches.

- Cut down or eliminate your caffeine consumption.

- If the overuse of regular pain relievers that contain caffeine is causing headaches, cut down on use and try natural methods of pain relief.

- If low blood sugar is causing your headaches, be sure to eat regular meals at regular times and to never skip a meal. See HYPOGLYCEMIA, page 243.

CHAPTER 32

Urinary Incontinence

Patricia was a virtual recluse by the time she came to see me. Like so many other women with urinary incontinence, she felt devastated by her inability to control her urine, and had severely curtailed many of her activities. She was in her mid-seventies, a short, apple-cheeked woman with gray hair and a clear complexion. She was visibly embarrassed when she walked into my office, and when I asked her to tell me about her problem she looked at me with something close to anguish.

"It started about a year ago," she said. "I noticed that sometimes, when I laughed too hard, or coughed, or made a sudden move, a few drops of urine would leak from my bladder. I didn't worry about it at first — I thought I might have an infection, or a cold. In fact, the doctor I went to see about it prescribed antibiotics — thinking it was due to an infection, you see. But it didn't clear up, it just got worse. Now it can happen suddenly, without warning, any time at all."

Patricia, like many of my other patients with urinary incontinence, had come to me for help while doubting that there could be any help for her condition. She felt isolated and ashamed, and seemed taken aback when I told her that urinary incontinence is quite common. Up to twenty million Americans suffer from urinary incontinence, most of them — but not all — elderly, and up to three-quarters of them women.

Sometimes the problem is caused by a bladder infection, and is accompanied by burning or irritation of the urethra during urination. The bladder infection, and related incontinence, will clear up with antibiotics. But, paradoxically, there are times when antibiotics or other medications are the cause of urinary incontinence. If you are on regular medications, ask your doctor if they could be contributing to the problem.

In Patricia's case there was no specific cause for the problem. Her doctor had told her there were medications that could control incontinence, but had warned her they would cause side effects, including dry mouth, eye problems, and a buildup of urine. Since there could be serious side effects from the medication, Patricia would have to remain under close medical supervision. She was willing to do it, she said, because anything was better than what she was going through — unless I had a natural therapy alternative. Was there a supplement, a vitamin she could take?

The Best Natural Approach To Urinary Incontinence

There are no known supplements that can cure urinary incontinence, but there is a simple exercise that has been enormously successful in controlling and often eliminating incontinence. It is called the Kegel exercise, and was developed in the 1940's to help pregnant women gain control over incontinence — caused when their enlarging uterus pressed down against the bladder. I described the exercises to Patricia, and told her about some basic guidelines to follow to help her control the problem that was confining her to her apartment.

Patricia seemed dubious that something as simple as the Kegel exercise could help, but she promised to try it when I assured her it had helped thousands of women. Three weeks later she called me to report guarded success. "It's beginning to work," she said, with a touch of wonder in her voice. "I've had a couple of accidents this week, but none at all for the last two days. I may be able to go to the Senior Center next week."

Urinary incontinence is the one medical condition no one wants to discuss — and it's a frequent reason for putting a loved one in a nursing home. So it's fortunate that the following guidelines have been so successful in clearing up the problem.

The Kegel Exercise

The Kegel exercise strengthens the muscles that surround the opening to the bladder. You can feel them by stopping the flow of urine during urination.

Here's how to do it. Three times or more each day:

1. Tense these muscles while slowly counting to four, and then release.
2. Repeat, continuing the exercise for at least two minutes.

You will start to notice a difference in about a week, and real results in three to four weeks. Don't stop doing the exercise once you regain control of your bladder — you must keep doing it to retain your muscular tone, or you will become incontinent again.

Avoid Aggravating Substances

There are substances that can irritate the bladder, such as smoke, caffeine, perfumes in soaps, bubble baths, and toiletries. Avoid anything that aggravates the problem.

Also, don't drink excessive amounts of fluids, which will stretch the bladder. Four glasses of fluids a day may be sufficient, unless there are medical reasons why you need to drink more.

The Right Amount Of Fluids

Some people who suffer from urinary incontinence begin to cut down on their fluid intake to the point where they begin to suffer from dehydration. Be sensible about fluid intake and check with your doctor if you are concerned about the amount of fluid you are drinking (either too much or too little), given your condition.

Don't allow your bladder to remain full. An overly full bladder becomes stretched out and prone to infection, and is, of course, more likely to leak. Void your bladder at least eight times during the day and, in particular, when you first get up, both before and after meals, and before going to bed.

The Cranberry Cure

Cranberry juice, which is acidic, is helpful in maintaining a healthy urinary system and should be a part of your daily diet. As many brands have too much sugar in them, try getting the cranberry juice at a health food store, and you may want to find one that is artificially sweetened.

For More Information. . .

A newsletter called "HIP: Help for Incontinent People," is put out by a non-profit, self-help organization. For a free copy, send a stamped, self-addressed envelope to HIP, Box 544, Union, S.C., 29379.

A Natural Treatment For Incontinence

- Check to see if any medications you take could be causing incontinence: check with your doctor and/or check the *Physicians' Desk Reference* at your library for a listing of side effects to prescription drugs.

- Kegel Exercise: Do this exercise every day, tightening your pelvic muscles for at least two minutes, three times a day or more.

- Avoid caffeine, alcohol, smoking, perfumes in soaps and bubble baths, toilet papers and feminine hygiene products.

- Drink cranberry juice.

- Unless there's a medical reason indicating otherwise, no more than four glasses of liquid daily are needed.

- Empty your bladder regularly, at least eight times a day.

CHAPTER 33

Vaginitis

Vaginitis is an inflammation of the vagina due to an infection or an irritating agent, which must be properly identified before it can be treated. Some women who suffer from recurring vaginitis don't realize it's due to a specific cause that be effectively treated.

Such was the case with Sandy, a woman in her mid-twenties who had been suffering from recurring vaginitis since she was in college. In Sandy's case, she proved to be allergic to the spermicide she and her boyfriend had been using. But I've also had patients who, having been infected by their boyfriend or husband, became reinfected after treatment.

To eradicate the infection once and for all, your sexual partner must also undergo treatment at the same time, or you'll continue a vicious cycle of infection. I've also seen patients who had chronic vaginitis because they were trying — unsuccessfully — to treat themselves for infection, or whose infection had been misdiagnosed by their doctor.

Most instances of infectious vaginitis are treated with presciption medication and must be diagnosed by a doctor. When the vaginitis is caused by an irritant or allergen, you might be able to detect — and eradicate — the cause yourself. To help you identify the problem and help you determine when to seek medical treatment, I've outlined the main causes of vaginitis.

Candida Albicans

Candida Albicans is the most common cause of vaginitis. Candida is a fungus that is always present in the vagina, but it starts to proliferate when certain physiological changes become conducive to its growth. The symptoms of a Candida infection are itching and a whitish, cheesy discharge. For additional information on the onset and treatment of CANDIDIASIS, please turn to page 115.

Trichomoniasis

Trichomoniasis is the next most common cause of vaginitis. Usually referred to as "trich," it is due to a protozoan introduced through sexual contact. Its symptoms are a greenish white or yellowish discharge with a foul odor. It is easily identified through a microscope, and treated with prescription medication.

A sexual partner must be treated at the same time to prevent reinfection.

Herpes

Herpes is a viral infection transmitted through sexual contact. Its symptoms, which occur two to eight days after contact with an infected partner, are very itchy, small, red bumps on the vulva, which develop into painful blisters and eventually burst. A man has similar symptoms on his genitals. A definitive diagnosis of herpes should be made by a doctor, who can also prescribe helpful medication. For additional information, please See HERPES, page 217.

Chlamydia

Chlamydia is the most frequent sexually-transmitted disease among young people in the United States, and can cause tubal scarring and infertility. If you are under twenty-five and are sexually active with multiple partners, there is a chance you have chlamydia. There are no symptoms until the disease is well advanced, though bleeding from the cervix upon swabbing by a doctor may be an indication of chlamydia. Pregnant women who have a vaginal infection should ask their doctor to test them for chlamydia, which can cause complications for the baby.

Gonorrhea

Gonorrhea is a sexually transmitted vaginal infection that should be treated immediately with antibiotics, as it can cause infertility if untreated.

Unfortunately, while there are obvious symptoms in a man — a noticeable discharge and painful urination — a woman may have no symptoms at all to tell her she's been infected. If you have reason to believe you might have been exposed to gonorrhea, ask your doctor do a diagnostic lab test, which will determine if you have been infected and should be treated.

Irritant Vaginitis

Irritant Vaginitis, is caused, as its name implies, by substances or activities irritating to the vagina. Ill-fitting diaphragms, or diaphragms and tampons left in too long will cause irritation. Detergents, douches, spermicides, latex condoms or soaps are examples of substances that may prove allergenic or irritating. And sexual activity without proper lubrication may prove irritating or traumatic. In this type of vaginitis, if you can identify the cause of the problem, you can take action to eliminate it or correct it without seeking medical advice.

Hormonal Vaginitis

Hormonal Vaginitis is caused by fluctuations in hormonal levels. The most common type of hormonal vaginitis is due to decreased hormonal activity, and is called "atrophic" vaginitis. It may be experienced by postmenopausal women and women who had their ovaries removed. Its symptoms are itching, burning, and a thin, watery discharge. If you believe you have this type of vaginitis, your doctor can prescribe topical or systemic hormones that will give you quick relief.

Increased vaginal discharge, quite common at the time of ovulation, is another cause for hormonal vaginitis. This is natural, and is not considered a medical problem. A warm water douche will help alleviate the condition.

Since the health of the vagina is closely connected to the health of your reproductive system and your overall health, it is important to correct problem conditions. As mentioned earlier, most vaginal infections will require medical attention. The following treatment will help you take the precautions necessary to insure a healthy bacterial level in the vagina, and prevent recurrence of infections.

A Natural Treatment For Candida And Trichomonas

As mentioned above, most vaginal infections will require the help of a gynecologist to treat and cure the condition. This is usually true of candida and trichomonas but, as they can recur in some women, I'm including here a list of precautions that can help prevent them. Most of these suggestions have to do with maintaining a healthy bacterial level in the vagina. (See CANDIDIASIS, page 115.)

- Do not wear tight pants or pantyhose. Excessive moisture invites infection. Cotton panties allow air to circulate and are preferable to nylon ones.
- Add the lactobacillus acidophilus culture to your diet. You can do this by eating a daily portion of yogurt which contains

live cultures — it must say so on the label — or by taking acidophilus capsules which are available in health food stores. I usually recommend 3 capsules daily.

- Betadine, an antibacterial agent available at pharmacies, is helpful in fighting vaginal infections including candida and trich. It kills most organisms within thirty seconds. Do not overuse this or any other douche; twice a day should be enough.

- Be sure to have your sexual partner treated along with you, especially if you have recurrent infections.

- If possible, discontinue sexual activity for the duration of your infection to reduce irritation to infected tissues and to avoid reinfection until you've completed treatment.

In addition to your daily basic antioxidant vitamin/mineral supplement, take:

- Vitamin C: 1000 mg. daily.
- Vitamin E: 400 I.U. daily.
- Beta-carotene: 25,000 I.U. daily.

CHAPTER 34

Varicose Veins

It's estimated that approximately 25 percent of American women suffer from varicose veins. It tends to be an inherited condition, aggravated by pregnancy, overweight, constipation, or lack of exercise. While varicose veins can be surgically removed, they tend to come back — unless you eliminate the aggregating factors that brought them on in the first place. That's what I explained to Diana, a patient who came in hoping I could tell her how to get rid of her varicose veins.

Diana, a teacher in her mid-thirties, was an attractive redhead who would have been even prettier if she had lost some thirty-odd pounds. She had recently become engaged to be married, and, as she planned the wedding and honeymoon in the Caribbean, she was mortified by the thought of herself at the beach, the prominent varicose veins on her legs exposed.

"Isn't there some vitamin, some supplement that will make them recede?" Diana wanted to know.

I told Diana that there were no supplements that would eradicate existing varicose veins. That could only be done surgically, or through a dermatological procedure that involves injecting a solution into the enlarged vein in order to have it collapse.

But there were several things she could do to prevent the onset of additional varicose veins and to improve the appearance of existing ones. While most women are primarily concerned about the cosmetic impact of varicose veins, it is their medical significance that should be the primary concern.

What Are Varicose Veins?

Varicose veins are a sign of stress on the circulatory system. When the circulatory system is placed under stress, whether from pregnancy, overweight, or constipation, the veins carrying blood back to the heart from the legs become engorged and dilated, and appear bluish and swollen.

As the veins weaken, there is a decrease of blood flow, and the capillaries may break, leaking fluid into the surrounding tissue. You will feel a tingling on the surface of your skin as the blood flow is reduced. You may notice small blue veins near the surface of the skin. Your legs may become swollen, and you may experience feelings of tightness and congestion in the veins. Your leg muscles may feel tired, and you may have muscular leg cramps.

If the condition becomes chronic, the skin may become ulcerated. In rare cases, complications of varicose veins may cause phlebitis, a condition where clots form on the wall of the vein, and pose the risk of traveling to the lungs with serious — and potentially fatal — results.

While Diana had some prominent veins on her legs, they had not deteriorated to the point of posing a medical problem. I urged Diana to keep them from deteriorating further by tackling the problems that had brought them on in the first place. My recommendations to Diana were the same as those for most of my patients who suffer from varicose veins: weight loss, a high fiber diet, and exercise.

Diana called just before the wedding to tell me she had lost twelve pounds and was still exercising and dieting. She had opted against having her varicose veins removed because they were so much less noticeable, she said. "As I lost weight, they became much less prominent, and I plan to use a self-tanning cream to camouflage them further."

Diana realized one of her problems was that, as a teacher, she had an essentially sedentary job which had her sitting at her desk or standing at the blackboard. Now, following my advice, she would stretch her legs by changing position, or walking down the length of the classroom. "It keeps my circulation going — and brings me closer to the kids," Diana remarked.

If you have varicose veins, or if you are predisposed to them because of a history of varicose veins in your family, these natural therapy guidelines will help you treat the problems that lead to, and aggravate, the condition.

> If varicose veins become a serious problem for you, either for cosmetic reasons or because of complications such as phlebitis, surgery may be indicated. Consult with your doctor.

Reduce Excess Weight

The more weight you carry, the more stress you place on your circulatory system. During pregnancy, when many women first develop varicose veins, the weight is temporary, and the situation is relieved immediately after birth. For anyone else who's carrying extra weight, weight reduction will provide relief to varicose veins.

Add Fiber To Your Diet

A high fiber diet is important for two reasons. First, it will help keep your weight under control. Secondly, it will help keep you from being constipated, which is one of the major causes of varicose veins. The stress of straining during a bowel movement puts great pressure on the veins, by obstructing the flow of blood up the legs and back to the heart. This stress results in varicose veins, and hemorrhoids as well. By promoting regular and easy bowel movements, a high fiber diet will be very helpful in relieving the stress that causes varicose veins.

Exercise

I urge all my patients with varicose veins to establish a program of regular aerobic exercise such as walking, running, or biking, all of which cause the calf muscles to contract and help push blood upwards through the veins. But such aerobic exercise is not enough. People with varicose veins should stretch their muscles frequently during the day, to keep the blood from pooling and engorging the veins. Just walking around your desk or kitchen counter every half-hour or so will be helpful. During a car trip, try to keep your legs elevated, as described below. When on a plane, you can take a walk down the aisle to give your legs a stretch.

Elevation And Support

When your legs are elevated higher than your hips, you are taking pressure off your circulatory system. Unless you work in your own office, you may not be able to put your feet on your desk, but you can certainly elevate your legs at home, while reading or watching television.

Some of my patients have also told me that elastic support stockings give them relief. These can be found in pharmacies and department stores, but the best ones are obtained in medical supply stores.

There's a trick to putting on elastic support hose. Or at least, there's a way to do it
that helps to make them more effective.

To put on your elastic support stockings:

1. Lie down on the floor next to a
   wall and, with your legs raised,
   place your feet against the wall.
   Stay in this position, which allows
   the blood to flow back towards
   the heart, for two or three minutes.
2. Slip on the stockings.

If you rest in this position a few times
each day you will relieve the pressure and
swelling in your legs.

Nutritional Supplements For Varicose Veins

I have found that Vitamin E is helpful for varicose veins.

Another helpful supplement is bioflavonoids,
which strengthen the capillaries and make it more
difficult for fluids to leak through. Studies have
shown that bioflavonoids help relieve leg fatigue
and heaviness, and my own patients have found
bioflavonoids helpful. A bioflavonoid called querce-

tin C, which comes from blue-green algae, has been found to be particularly effective.

If you take quercetin C, you don't have to take additional bioflavonoids.

Spider Alert

If you noticed that you developed spider veins after you began to take birth control pills, you should know that sometimes these veins develop as a result of hormonal imbalance. Consult your doctor.

A Natural Treatment For Varicose Veins

- Keep weight at appropriate level avoiding obesity.
- Adopt a high fiber diet including plentiful fresh fruits, vegetables, and whole grains. Use bulking agents as needed (see CONSTIPATION page 143).
- Exercise: Regular "major" exercise to contract the leg muscles, especially running, walking, cycling. Regular "minor" exercise as a relief from sitting or standing for long periods of time, such as stretching the legs or briefly walking.

In addition to your daily basic antioxidant vitamin/mineral, take:

- Vitamin E: 400 I.U. daily.
- Bioflavonoids: 1000 to 2000 mg. daily. Or take:
  - Quercitin-C: 100 mg. three times daily.

Also

- Elevate your legs — ideally with your ankles higher than your hips — whenever possible.
- Wear support stockings, preferably fitted and from a medical supply house. Lie on back with hips near wall and legs perpendicular to floor to encourage blood flow. Rest in this position for a few minutes before putting on stockings.

CHAPTER 35

Wrinkle Prevention

The cosmetic industry is a multi-billion dollar industry and getting larger each year. But, while there are excellent products available, you need more than creams and cosmetics to retain a supple, healthy skin. Your skin is your largest organ, the outside reflection of your overall health. It is of diagnostic value for your doctor, who can tell a lot about your health by the texture, color, and temperature of your skin.

Good nutrition, exercise, and sufficient sleep are the best ways to insure a healthy, supple skin, which is why many movie actors and models insist on getting eight hours of sleep. The healthier you are, the better your skin will look.

There are also a number of precautions you can take to protect your skin:

Drink Sufficient Fluids

Many of my patients don't realize that one of the primary functions of the skin is to excrete toxins from the body. To dilute the negative effects of these toxins, which may produce rashes and leave your skin feeling dry and dull, I recommend eight glasses of water a day.

Sunscreen Is Critical

Skin doesn't wrinkle because of age. Skin wrinkles because of the sun. Quite elderly women still normally have beautiful skin along their breasts and on the inside of their arms, where the sun has not scorched it over the decades. Keep in mind that the harmful effects of the sun can be damaging even on a cloudy day.

To protect your face from the effects of the sun, put on sunscreen right after your morning shower all year long — summer and winter. If your makeup or daytime moisturizer includes sunscreen, make sure that it's at least SPF 15 or above.

Many people have had allergic reactions to a sunscreen ingredient called PABA, and most manufacturers have stopped using it in their products. If you break out in a rash, check to see if your sunscreen contains PABA. Whether it does or not, discontinue using it, and test the next sunscreen on your arm before putting it on your face.

When you're planning an outdoor activity such as golf, tennis, swimming or bicycle riding, apply your sunscreen half an hour before you start, to give it time to work, and then reapply it regularly. Keep in mind that skin cancer rates have shot up alarmingly, and that the results of sun damage are cumulative and can be truly frightening. With the improved sunscreens available on the market, you can enjoy all outdoor sports and still protect your skin from sunburn.

Stop Smoking

Smoking ages your skin prematurely, and if you smoke a pack and a half a day, you'll wrinkle ten years earlier than your non-smoking twin. Nicotine, which constricts blood vessels and interferes with the flow of nutrients, has a drying, caustic effect on the system. In addition, just the act of pursing your lips to inhale and exhale will, over a period of time, etch prune-like wrinkles around your lips, while the smoke that blows around your face is going to dry it out.

Use A Moisturizer

People with oily skin wrinkle less than people with dry skin because their skin is lubricated. If you have dry, or "combination" skin — part dry and part oily — use moisturizer daily to keep your skin lubricated. See also DRY SKIN, page 181.

Nutritional Supplements For The Skin

Vitamins A and C are both excellent for the health of your skin, and should be taken daily.

A Natural Treatment For
Wrinkle Prevention

- Drink six to eight eight-ounce glasses of water each day.
- *Always* use a sunscreen with an SPF of 15 or higher, not just when you're at the beach. Apply it each day before you leave the house and reapply it at midday.
- Stop smoking.
- Moisturize your skin (see DRY SKIN, page 181).

In addition to your daily basic antioxidant vitamin/ mineral, take:

- Vitamin C: 1000 mg. daily.
- Vitamin A: 10,000 to 25,000 I.U. daily.

A Final Word From Doctor Giller

Have you ever felt as if your doctor ignored everything you said? Well, you're not alone.

A recent study revealed that doctors are twice as likely to dismiss a woman's symptoms and declare "they're all in your head." That means they're *twice* as likely to ignore a serious condition . . . *just because you're a woman!*

It's not fair. It's downright *dangerous*. But it's true.

And did you know that heart disease is the *number one* killer of women . . . yet nearly all the heart disease research has been done on *men?*

Just look at these five examples from **Outrageous Practices** by Leslie Laurence and Beth Weinhouse (Fawcett-Columbine, 1994):

- The landmark study that revealed how aspirin can help prevent heart attacks was performed on 22,000 men only. Page 4.
- A Harvard study of the links between caffeine and heart disease tracked 45,000 men and not a single woman! Page 61.
- A major study of the links between heart disease and high cholesterol was performed on 13,000 men. Women were deliberately excluded from the study. Page 61.

And It Gets Worse . . .

- Did you know that no conclusive, scientific research has ever been performed concerning the long-term safety of birth control pills?
- And has anyone told you that women with kidney failure are 30 percent less likely to get a life-saving kidney transplant?

Why are women being ignored by the medical establishment?

Because many researchers believe a woman's hormones can "slant" the results. Because they believe women are too "emotional" when reporting their symptoms. And because it would be "too expensive" to test *both* men and women.

In my opinion, this blatant neglect of women and their unique healthcare needs represents an appalling injustice.

Why? Because it means there are millions of doctors who have been trained to *ignore* what you say. It means that you're given "hand-me-down" healthcare based on research performed on *men* only. And most dangerous of all, it severely limits your healthcare options.

You deserve to know about *all* your healing choices. If there's a safer alternative to the "drugs and surgery" approach favored by most doctors, don't you deserve to know about it? If there's a *natural* remedy that will treat the *root cause* of your problem (instead of just "masking" the symptoms), shouldn't you try that first?

Of course you should! But you'll almost never hear about these options from the medical establishment. That's why I have made it my life's work to find safe, *natural* prescriptions that work where drugs and surgery fail.

And now I'm delighted to say that, with this book, *Natural Prescriptions For Women*, I am going public with my best, safest natural prescriptions. I know that no single book can possibly compensate for the years of neglect the medical establishment has shown for women. But this new book is overflowing with natural cures that work.

For twenty years, I have used these prescriptions for myself and my patients . . . and achieved almost unbelievable healing. These are not "quack" cures.

They are the real thing. And they are proven safe and almost 100 percent *effective*.

It is my sincerest hope that you will use them to repair and restore your health . . . and avoid the dangerous trap of drugs and surgery.

Yours truly,

Robert M. Giller, M.D.

About the Authors

Robert M. Giller, M.D.

Robert M. Giller, M.D. trained in internal medicine at the University of Illinois and New York Hospital. During his term of duty in the army, he specialized in preventive medicine and public health, which laid the groundwork for his long interest in the preventive and alternative medicine field. Dr. Giller is a member of the College of Preventive Medicine and a Fellow of the American Academy of Family Practice.

Dr. Giller, with Kathy Matthews, is the author of the bestsellers *Medical Makeover, Maximum Metabolism* and *Natural Prescriptions*. He hosts a popular radio program on WOR, "In the Doctor's Office," reaching listeners from Boston to Philadelphia. He lives in New York City.

Kathy Matthews

Kathy Matthews is a writer specializing in medical subjects. In addition to Dr. Giller's books, she has co-authored nine other books, including *Nutripoints* with Roy Vartabedian, *On Women and Beauty* with Sophia Loren and *Christie Brinkley's Complete Outdoor Fitness and Beauty Book* with Christie Brinkley.

Index

A

Accutane, 47
Acetaminophen, 105–106, 334
Acidophilus, 13, 118, 119, 120,
    157, 223–224, 349, 350
Acne, 41–51, 131, 316
Acupressure points, 300, 301
Acupuncture, 12, 74, 106, 124
Aging, 33
Alcohol, 29–30, 59, 64, 85, 88,
    92, 98, 119, 157, 163,
    213, 234, 241, 250, 251,
    252, 256, 257, 258, 304,
    308, 309, 310, 318, 344
Allergies, 35, 36, 44, 45, 46, 49,
    50, 58, 62, 116, 119,
    164, 167, 171, 181, 182,
    185, 187, 188, 190–191,
    195, 201, 202, 203, 285,
    290, 321, 322, 335, 337,
    345, 346, 348, 360
Aloe vera, 149, 150
Aluminum, 148
Alzheimer's disease, 271
Anemia, 207, 208
Angina, 53–65, 95
Antioxidants, 33, 34, 36, 37,
    46, 47, 59, 76, 95, 96
Arginine, 223, 225
Arthritis, 14, 58, 67–81, 111,
    112, 122, 161, 304

Aspartame, 74, 75, 80, 284,
    288
Aspirin, 14, 62, 64, 68, 71, 72,
    102, 105, 203, 207, 208,
    288, 289, 291, 334, 364
Asthma, 28, 190, 304
Atherosclerosis, 38, 55, 83–99,
    136, 278

B

Back pain, 101–113, 152, 316
Bag Balm, 185, 188
Benson, Dr. Herbert, 261, 326,
    327, 328
Benzoyl peroxide, 48, 49
Beta-carotene, 32, 33, 34, 57,
    59, 60, 61, 63, 95, 96,
    98, 131, 132, 138, 139,
    141, 194, 195, 222, 350
Bethesda system, 128, 130
Bioflavonoids, 155, 157, 207,
    208, 224, 356, 357, 358
Black currant seed oil, 48
Blackheads, 43, 49
Bladder, 153, 154, 155, 157,
    269, 339
  infections, 116, 151
Blood pressure, 28, 57, 59, 62,
    64, 92, 93, 94, 96, 136,
    161, 227, 228, 229, 230,